The Celtic Diet

The Celtic Diet

Let History Shape Your Future

Breanne Findlay

Order this book online at www.trafford.com
or email orders@trafford.com

Most Trafford titles are also available at major online book retailers.

Printed in the United States of America.

ISBN: 978-1-4669-6357-3 (sc)
ISBN: 978-1-4669-6356-6 (e)

Trafford rev. 10/25/2012

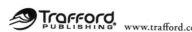 www.trafford.com

North America & international
toll-free: 1 888 232 4444 (USA & Canada)
phone: 250 383 6864 ♦ fax: 812 355 4082

Dedicated to:

Dandy, my Grandmother, Helen Davidson Findlay

Pops, my Grandfather, Archibald Bunting Findlay

and James Robert Findlay, my Dad

Table of Contents

Introduction

Science and technology have made staggering contributions to our lives over the past five decades, such as medical breakthroughs, satellite communications, computers, contact lenses, Kevlar, bank machines, domestic printers, MRI's, Walkmans, Windows, HD TV, fuel cells, space stations, You Tube . . . and the list goes on.

Yet, some of the things made high tech should have left alone. I'm referring to our agriculture and our food, the basics we need every single day in order to ensure a healthy life.

The Celtic Diet is a no-nonsense, health inducing approach to a sound lifestyle, with whole grains, fruits, vegetables, fish, meat and un-processed foods. The Celtic Diet is also a simple, easy and inexpensive way to achieve your health goal.

Food items that you consume everyday will be put to you in a different way. In truth, back to the way it was. Discover these logical yet simple methodologies that will add simplicity to your eating habits while increasing your health and decreasing your waistline. You will see how adding whole grain oats will allow for numerous health benefits, benefits that you will feel virtually instantly.

The Celts were a resilient group, withstanding decades and even centuries of living hard and working hard. When the new world was open to those who were looking for a new life, or a new adventure, the Celts were durable, strong and healthy enough to withstand the treacherous voyage to North America. Here they started fresh lives, bringing with them the seeds and plants that they would need to continue their healthy ways. People that thrived on this diet built the new world.

We are taking the old basics and adding natural new components, where together, we will see the synergy of traditional and contemporary combine to make us healthy again.

The Celtic Diet is traditionally based, contemporarily recreated, scientifically proven, medically accepting, physically welcoming, financially inexpensive, spiritually sound, and historically verified. Let a large history shape you into a thinner future.

Why we must eat simpler

In 1992, President George H. W. Bush made an Executive Order that foods that are genetically modified or genetically engineered DO NOT have to be disclosed on any labeling. There is an international organization called the Codex Alimentarius, where countries met to discuss that such labeling be made mandatory. All countries but the United States.

Under this Executive Order, modified foods are not required to undergo any safety testing before entering the market. Suggesting that the FDA has already ensured that any mutated foods grown in the future are pre-approved to be safe.

Today, approximately 80% of all foods have been genetically altered. Unfortunately, we don't know which ones. Some major points were made at this meeting. Some of these sounding like they came out of a Frankenstein movie. In short, these concerns are:

1. that those with personal and religious beliefs towards their foods will be unknowingly consuming the product or food group they wish to avoid. For example, corn that was modified with a gene from pigs would not be wanted by Vegetarians, kosher Jews or Halal Muslims. Also, Jewish and Christian believers of God creating heaven, earth and all living creatures, would want to avoid non-God made foods;

2. unknown future effects, example being that animals fed corn with a spermicide modification were becoming sterile, with the same fear that human males will suffer the same;

3. in Russia, GM soya that were fed to female rats produced stunted pups, with over half dying in three weeks. This experiment was repeated with the same results. The surviving pups were sterile;

4. 1000's of sheep in India died while grazing on bacteria-treated crops;

5. antibodies from a Monsanto company altered corn hybrid flowered, subsequently injured people from the toxic Bt protein;

6. horses consuming similar modified corn had to be put down after contracting mysterious diseases;

7. that GM soya negatively affected the pancreatic, hepatic liver and testicular cells in mice;

8. damage to every organ in the systems of rats that were fed GM potatoes;

9. chicken fed GM corn were 200% more likely to die prematurely.

There is no proof that these modified plants carry the same nutritional equivalent of naturally grown plants. Therefore the nutrients could be genetically modified as well and be unsafe to eat.

Farm workers that have handled GM produce have broken out in skin conditions, thus showing that consumers need to know about the risks with GM foods. Also, some countries state that inadequate labelling of mutated foods equates to human experimentation without consent, according to the Nuremberg Code.

Fact is, our food is becoming less food-like in the hands of corporations. And these aren't necessarily food companies, these corporations are chemical companies that have devised methods to control the agriculture in the US. Chemical engineers don't belong in our food.

Celtic History

Sometimes a new concept in a healthy eating plan originates from the past. Let's learn a little history about the Celtic Culture.

The People

'Celtic' refers to a number of European people who speak the Celtic Languages, some of which being Irish, Scottish, Gaelic, Manx, Welsh and Cornish. All stemming from the cultures of Ireland, Scotland, Wales, Cornwall, the Isle of Man and Brittany.

Today, the term 'Celt' or 'Celtic" is used for those that speak one of the Celtic languages **and** their descendants, but has also been used in team sports names such as the Boston Celtics and the Celtic Football Club. Galacia and Asturias, both self governed sections of Spain are sometimes considered a Celtic nation due to their historic traditions and naming practices, yet neither speak any of the Celtic languages. England retains some Celtic influences, but again no Celtic language. France too is associated with the Celts as they share historic roots to the Gauls of western Europe.

At the present time, Celtic culture is visible in many parts of this multicultural world. People with family roots in Europe will have a Celtic connection of some sort. The ancient Celtic culture still thrives in the modern world through art, music, writing and spirituality. It is the early literature in the Welsh and Irish languages that has help preserve the Celtic beliefs that nature, spirituality and the material world synergistically combine.

The Celts are thought to have their beginnings in central Europe, now known as Germany, Austria, Slovakis, the Czech Republic and Hungary. From there, these peoples expanded across the continent, inhabiting a much larger portion of Europe.

There were two main Celtic groups. One being the 'lowland Celts' from the Danube who were skilled in metalwork and considered agriculturally advanced, blending in peacefully with other cultures while they settled and slowly spread westwards. Their religious beliefs included a predominately matriarchal society.

The second group, sometimes referred to as the 'true' Celts, was still quite similar to the lowland group, living on the Rhine in sixth century BC. Originating from the Balkans and Carpathians as a militarily aristocracy and fighting their way through Rome and Delphi. In seemingly opposition to their aggressive qualities, they had a great sensitivity to music, poetry and philosophy.

The name Celt originated from the ancient Greek word "keltoi". Being a broad and culturally linguistic group, they were a collection of tribal nations, never being a single empire and ruled by one government.

There is not an abundance of information on the elusive culture of the Celts. What we do know is from ancient documents, one written by Herodotus, a Roman writer. To the orderly Roman Empire, the Celts appeared barbarous and primitive. Archaeology has proven that the Celtic culture was powerful and complex and has had a large impact on numerous civilizations for centuries. The possibly first archaeological evidence originates from what is now France and Germany, dating back to the Bronze Age, approximately 1200 BC. It is presumed the Celts settled in the now known British Isles in around 900 to 700 BC, and continued their settlements from 600 to 200 BC in the Black Sea area.

Around 500 BC, the Celts expanded into Italy, Macedonia and Thessalia taking over portions of Rome. Eventually the Romans subdued the Celts, and most of Britain was under the Roman Empire. Meanwhile, the Celtic culture was surviving in France, Wales, Scotland and Ireland. The Celtic tribes were united by a common speech, customs and practices, and their economy was governed by an agricultural life. Here their lives were working the land and tending to livestock.

The Celts religion was previously known as Druidism. Celtic tradition was abounding with Pagan beliefs including deities of the earth, woodland spirits, sun gods, fertility gods and goddesses, and many animals were seen as sacred. Many festivals and events can be attributed to the ancient Celtic traditions, such as Halloween.

The Celts respected the earth, believing that the Avon River had healing powers and honored the great oak tree.

The art and architecture of the Celts was widespread and diverse, and today is still considered one of the first great contributions to European art as a whole. Influenced by ancient Persian, Etruscan, Greek, Roman and Scythian art, yet retaining a style of its own.

With a respect for the earth, animals and plants were often found depicted, more often than any human representation.

Celtic Knot work is well known for its highly sophisticated and geometric patterns, balancing curves and spirals in harmonious designs. These styles of art designs were placed on objects such as weapons, household items, statues and jewelery. Wood and stone was also used to carve large and intricate pieces.

In the first century AD, the Romans conquered the British Isles and realized the Celtic beliefs were similar to the old Roman religion. It was these beliefs that assisted in the alliance of the Greeks and the Romans, who saw a correlation between religions and this was used to create an emergence of cultures, especially through the water of Avon, which the Romans also believed to have healing powers.

Most of us were probably not aware of all the contributions from the Celtic cultures of past. From St. Patrick's Day to plaid designs and whisky. The word "Celtic" itself is used in a variety a topics.

The Food

In the prehistoric United Kingdom area, the peoples then would have ate whale, seal, fish, shellfish, sea birds (including geese and ducks), and game animals such as deer, wild pig, elk, wild ox, bear and beaver. Around 3,500 years ago (or 1,500 BC) came sheep, goats, cattle, and pigs, all of which were eaten and used for other products such as milk, wool, etc.

If you take Celts in Roman and post-Roman Britain they had fish, shellfish, deer, boar, hares, wild fowl. The Romans introduced what was termed "delicate birds" such as pheasants, peacocks, pigeons and guinea fowl. Cattle were exported to the continent before the Romans arrived. There is also historic mentioning of veal and beef with sauces, ham and bacon, much mutton, and goats. There is some evidence horse meat was eaten, at least in sausages, as well as domestic fowl.

Irish foods of the approximate same time period, included boiled bacon with kale or cabbage, which is what was eaten in Ireland before Americans imported a variant on the New England Boiled Dinner (corned beef and cabbage, with separately boiled potatoes, but no traditional beets), sometime during the late 1800's to early 1900's. Kale or cabbage boiled with salt pork, ham, or bacon is a standard porrey or joutes dish, found in periodic sources from France, England, and Germany. Le Menagier gives several such recipes, while Taillevent doesn't bother, since, he says, "every housewife already knows how to make them". It can safely be presumed this dish was eaten in Ireland in pre-history.

In some archaeological digs, dating back to the 1300's, the analysis of samples from the Dublin area indicate that of the meat that was eaten, 90% was from mature cattle (beef not veal), 7% from young pigs and the remaining 3% from sheep or goats. Horse was also occasionally eaten as were dogs, cats, deer, seals and whales.

Additionally, they have identified the remains of crushed hens eggs, and all beef would have been grass fed—not GM corn fed like today.

All in all, the foods identified were:

Grains and pulses identified included oats, barley, rye, wheat and peas (always dried versions);

Fruits and nuts: hazelnut, hawthorn, fig, strawberry, walnut, apple, sour cherry, plum, sloe, rose hip, blackberry, raspberry, elder, rowan, frochan/bilberry and grape. The fig and grape were imports and found listed in a 13th century shipping log book.

Other edible plants include wild celery, the Brassica sp.'s (turnip, cabbage, radish, brussel sprouts, etc.), black mustard, wild carrot, fennel and nettle. Potatoes were introduced in the 1600's.

Poultry and game, included rabbit, hare, turtle, goose, duck, partridge and quail. Pheasant would have originated in Asia, turkey from America, and Guinea fowl from Africa.

Fish and shellfish, which included mussels, cockles, scallops and oysters, along with trout, salmon and herring.

Cooking methods were not always mentioned. Roasting and baking would have been more common with the upper classes. Meat pieces in a stew can go a lot further than being roasted whole. Same goes for breads, most people not being the upper class would have fried their breads or baked them on a bake stone beside the fire. Many frying pan types of cookware have been discovered at these sites. Yet the boiling of meats is well mentioned in historic texts.

Most meals would have been some form of stew, soup or pottage cooked in a cauldron over the central hearth of the house. Bread, baked in a clay oven or on a griddle, would also be a daily fare. Flour could be ground at a water mill although more usually it would be done in the home using a hand quern. Wealthier people would have been able to afford an imported rotary quern from the Rhineland.

When the flour is freshly querned from recently cut grain, little yeast is necessary to be added to the dough as there is a reasonable yeast content in fresh grain.

Food was eaten from wooden or clay bowls using only a knife and spoon (forks do not seem to have been used for eating until much later in the medieval period). There are however, Scandinavian finds of pointed 'food sticks' made of wood or bone which may have been used for picking up pieces of meat and larger vegetables. Wooden plates were used for some food and pottery ones were very rare. Drinking vessels were made from a variety of materials in a number of styles. The most common would have been wooden or pottery cups and mugs. Horns (often highly decorated) were also used and conical glass vessels were used in the early period, but were rare, giving way to glass vessels shaped more like beakers that we have today. Small wooden cups were used for very strong drinks. Leather was also used for drinking vessels although there is little evidence of this other than a passage in Ælfrics Colloquy. There is no evidence for drinking vessels with handles ever being used. Drinks were served from pottery jugs and pitchers or from bottles made of wood, clay or leather. Wooden tubs and ladles were probably used for serving drinks, some of which were served hot.

Alcohol

I would never suggest that anyone consume alcohol, especially as part of a healthy eating plan, but any historical tour of the Celtic Nations would be at a loss if there were no mention of the ales and alcohols that were created. You won't find any recipes that include these ingredients nor will you find them listed as part of your daily dietary plan.

Although the monks originally considered whisky to have medicinal value we know now that this isn't necessarily an accurate assessment of alcohol. Even myself, not being a drinker, would feel gladly obligated, for purely academic reasons, to sample the variety of historically made drinks. These particular alcohols would have been made in small batches and with organic ingredients.

Ale

A building dating back 5,000 years, (3000 BC), was uncovered in Skara Brae, Scotland and from the artifacts found, thought to have been a brewery. In those days, various north European tribes including the Celts and the Picts, made ale from malted spelt and flavoured it with the medicinal herb Meadowsweet. Bittering herbs like Meadowsweet were used to flavor and preserve ale, and perhaps add additional pain relieving properties as Meadowsweet contains salicin, a more stomach-friendly alternative to salicylic acid from willow bark. Thomas Pennant wrote in 'A Tour in Scotland' in 1769, that "ale is frequently made of the young tops of heath, mixing two thirds of that plant with one of malt, sometimes adding hops".

Scotland continued creating ales with herbs longer than the British did, but by the end of the 1800's, hops replaced herbs in Scottish brewing methods as well. One hundred years later, in 1990, the use of bittering herbs in ale was revived and can be found in Scotland today.

Throughout Europe, the brewing techniques were generally the same. 'Alewives' aka 'broustaris' in monasteries were what we would call brew masters. In 1509 in Aberdeen, there were 150 brewers and all women, while in London, 60% of the 290 brewers were women. In 1342, the Brewers' Guild in London was formed and later in 1598 the Edinburgh Society of Brewers.

In 1707, the 'Acts of Union' that were held in England, inadvertently gave Scottish breweries a significant financial advantage. Taxes on beer were lower than the rest of the United Kingdom and there were no taxes on malt in Scotland. This lead to numerous large and future famous Scottish brewers to be established and gave serious competition to other brewers worldwide. By 1850, the Edinburgh brewers were acknowledged as one of the foremost brewing centers in the world.

The Edinburgh brewers enjoyed quite a success with their strong hoppy ales, with exports to India, the British Empire, Russia, British Colonies and America. Some believe that the hard well water of Edinburgh contributes to these ale's successes. Some also believed that the Scottish brewers used less hops than their British counterparts, but historic records indicated that they used virtually the same amount, being 1.8 oz of hops per imperial gallon. These hoppy ales had become known by two different names, the British version was called a pale ale and the Scottish version called a Scotch ale.

Drambuie

Drambuie is an 80 proof traditional golden scotch whisky liqueur made from aged malt whisky, heather honey and a secret blend of herbs and spices. In 1746, exiled Prince Charles Edward Stuart was given sanctuary by Scottish Captain John Mackinnon. For his safe accommodation, Prince Stuart gave the Drambuie recipe to Captain Mackinnon, whose family has produced this prized liquor ever since. The name Drambuie (officially named in 1893) comes for the Scottish Gaelic phrase 'an dram buidheach' which means the 'drink that satisfies'.

Although Drambuie is a whisky liqueur, it has a very different flavour to Scotch Whisky due to the addition of heather and herbs. Produced in Scotland, on the Isle of Skye, the first commercial distribution of Drambuie occurred, with a mere twelve cases, in 1910.

Scotch Whisky

Scotch Whisky, generally known as Scotch in English speaking countries, and as Whisky in Scotland, can be made anywhere in the world but it cannot carry the word Scotch in its name. Legally, true Scotch Whisky can only be made in Scotland. It must be made from water and malted barley, to which other whole grains may be added. Oak casks are used for maturation, aged for no less than three years and a day.

We do know that the monks brought their distillation practices with them in approximately 400 AD. The political unrest toward the monasteries contributed to this since many of the monks, driven from their sanctuaries, had no choice but to put their skills to use. One of the first recorded financial documentations is where "Eight bolls of malt to Friar John Cor wherewith to make aqua vitae" (water of life). This was sufficient to produce almost 1500 bottles, and indicates that distilling was already a well-established practice. The first taxes on whisky production were ordered in 1644, causing an increase in underground or illegal distilleries. In 1780 there were approximately 8 legal operations to 400 not-legal ones. Parliament knew that it was losing a lot of taxes or income on this product, so in 1823 they eased restrictions on operating a distillery allowing for the flourishing of this industry.

Types of whisky include Malt Whisky (or single malt whisky) that contains no other grain than malted barley and distilled in pot stills. Grain Whisky (or single grain whisky) may contain unmalted barley and other malted or unmalted grains such as wheat and corn. The 'single' designation in this title refers to the fact that this whisky is made at one distillery only. At present there are dozens or malt whisky distilleries yet only seven grain distilleries, most located in the Scottish Lowlands.

Salts, Herbs and Spices

In the Celtic days, herbs were considered a vegetable and thus given much importance in the daily preparation of food. Herbs and spices are truly the saving grace in making flavourful meals. Most herbs can become an aromatic cup of tea, and spices will bring a plain soup to a gourmet status. The recipes in the following pages should be mere guidelines when creating your healthy meals, let your imagination and personal flavor favorites dictate your exclusive recipes.

Parsley

The two most popular types of parsley are Curly Parsley and Italian Flat Leaf Parsley which is more fragrant and less bitter. While parsley is a wonderfully nutritious and healing food, it is often under-appreciated. Most people do not realize that this plant has more uses than just being a decorative garnish that accompanies restaurant meals. Parsley is actually a warehouse of nutrients.

In the 1800's, Parsley was brought to the Celtic culture through the ancient trade routes from Sardinia. Cultivated for over 2,000 years, the world's most popular herb was used medicinally before becoming a food source. It's name means 'rock celery' and once established this biennial will return to your garden every year.

Parsley contains two unusual components that provide unique health benefits. The first component is volatile oil, which includes myristicin, limonene, eugenol, and alpha-thuiene. The activity of parsley's volatile oils qualify it as a 'chemo-protective' food, with potent anti-oxidant abilities, helping to neutralize some carcinogens such as benzopyrenes from cigarette smoke. The second component is flavonoids, which includes apiin, apigenin, crisoeriol, and luteolin. Luteolin, in particular, shows superior anti-oxidant activity by combining with oxygen-full molecules and preventing damage to oxygen based cells. Extracts of parsley have increased the anti-oxidant capacity of blood and is a source of nutrients to protect cardiovascular function.

Three vital nutrients that parsley is excellent for is Vitamin C, beta-carotene, and folic acid. Vitamin C is our body's primary water-soluble antioxidant, neutralizing dangerous free radicals. It is these free radicals that aid to the development and progression of numerous diseases and conditions, such as arteriosclerosis, colon cancer, diabetes, and asthma. People who consume Vitamin C rich foods have reduced risks for these ailments while promoting a healthy immune system that will fight infections. Osteoarthritis and rheumatoid arthritis symptoms have known to decrease due to it's anti-inflammatory powers.

The anti-oxidant, beta-carotene, works in the fat-soluble areas of our bodies. Beta-carotene rich foods are related to a reduction in the development of arteriosclerosis, diabetes, and cancer, and reducing the severity of asthma, osteoarthritis and rheumatoid arthritis. Vitamin A, the 'anti-infection vitamin', is a converted element from beta-carotene and a nutrient seriously needed for a strong immune system.

Folic Acid is a crucial B vitamin that assists in cardiovascular health. Folic Acid converts dangerous homocysteine molecules into benign molecules. Homocysteine can damage blood vessels; increase risk of heart attack and/or stroke. Folic Acid is needed for proper cell division and vital for cancer prevention, notably in the two areas that contain rapidly dividing cells, those being the colon and the cervix.

In the Annals of the Rheumatic Diseases, 2004, findings were concluded from a study of over 20,000 subjects who at the start were arthritis free. Of the subjects that developed arthritis, their food journals showed that they consumed the lowest amount of Vitamin C rich foods. These subjects were three times more likely to develop arthritis that those who consumed the highest amounts of Vitamin C.

Other medicinal uses include parsley tea as a diuretic. Chinese and German herbalogists recommend parsley tea to help control high blood pressure, and the Cherokee Nation use it as a tonic to strengthen the bladder. It is also often used as an emmenagogue to promote menstruation. Parsley appears to increase diuresis by enhancing sodium and water excretion while increasing potassium reabsorption.

Sage

There are hundreds of varieties of Sage, aka Salvia, the most common being Salvia Officinalis. Common Sage has pointed grey-green velvety leaves with deep veining and a pungent aroma. It can grow to a height of over 2 feet with pink, purple or white flowers. A member of the mint family, sage was not used as a food flavoring until the 1600's. In 1597 the herbalist John Gerard said that it was "singularly good for the head and quickeneth the nerves and memory." Sage has a reputation for restoring failing memory in the elderly and like other memory-enhancing herbs it has been traditionally associated with longevity.

Historically, when the British started importing tea from China, the Chinese would trade two cases of tea for one case of dried English sage. The leaves and stems are used in cooking for flavoring sausages, pork, sauces, cheese, dressings and stuffing as well as for tea.

Sage is among the best herbal choices for killing bacteria, but it is also amazing for culinary uses. Sage is a wonderful perennial herb for your garden. It's uses continue to grow, from its oils for aromatherapy to cooking and medicinal teas, and as well as its appearance in a garden.

Coriander

Coriander and Cilantro are named for different parts of the same herb. Coriander is the seed that is sometimes used in place of caraway seeds and cilantro is considered the leaves.

The leaves may be referred to coriander leaves, cilantro, Chinese parsley or Mexican parsley and the leaves do taste different from the seeds, being similar to juicier, citrus-like parsley.

Coriander's medicinal properties include having the ability to clear the body of lead, aluminium and mercury as well as being able to exhibit antibacterial action against E. Coli. and salmonella. Research is showing more benefits such as the relief of anxiety and insomnia, having 'anti-diabetic' properties, being an antiinflammatory and cholesterol lowering.

Coriander is mentioned in Exodus and it's cultivation has been confirmed in an archaeological event dating from the Early Bronze Age. Much used in our medieval Celtic cuisine due to its ability to make spoiled meats edible by covering rotten odors, (although I would not suggest doing that) and is still an important ingredient in sausage products.

Coriander is one of the first spices cultivated by early settlers having been brought with the Celtic settlers in North America in 1670.

Here is a traditional recipe for Cormarye, a spice blend for roasting meat:

> *"Take colyaundre, caraway smale grounded, powdour of peper and garlec ygrounde, in rede wyne; medle alle thise togyder and salt it. Take loynes of pork rawe and fle of the skyn, and pryk it wel with a knyf, and lay it in the sawse. Roost whan thou wilt, & kepe that that fallith therfro in the rostyng and seeth it in a possynet with faire broth, & serve it forth with the roost anoon."*

Translation: Take coriander, caraway seeds, ground pepper, ground garlic and mix with salt in a cup of red wine. Take pork loins with no skin, tenderize it and place in the red wine sauce. Roast when you like and keep the drippings for a gravy and serve it with roasted onions.

Mustard Seed

The Mustard Plant belongs to the Brassica family of cruciferous plants such as broccoli and cabbage. Like the other cruciferous plants, mustard seeds contain high amounts of phytonutrients and are repeatedly studied for their anti-cancer effects. To date there is evidence of the inhibition of existing cancer cell growth and protection from the formation of cancer cells.

Mustard seeds contain: selenium, omega-3 fatty acids, phosphorous, magnesium, manganese, dietary fiber, iron, calcium, protein, niacin and zinc. Selenium is a nutrient that can help reduce asthma and decrease rheumatoid arthritis symptoms. Magnesium can reduce asthma as well, lower high blood pressure, restore normal sleep patterns from menopausal symptoms, reduce migraines, and prevent atherosclerosis-related heart attacks.

Historically, Mustard Seeds were mentioned in the bible and in the ancient Sanskrit writings of 3000 BC. These amazing seeds are one of the most popular spices traded in the world, growing well in temperate climates including the Celtic countries, Canada and the United States.

Basic Mustard Recipe

1/3 cup mustard seeds

1/3 cup cider vinegar

1/2 clove garlic

3 T water

3 T honey

1/4 tsp sea salt

Combine mustard seeds, vinegar and garlic in a covered bowl and refrigerate for 36 hours. Remove and discard garlic and grind with water until blended but coarse, add honey and sea salt. Jar and refrigerate.

Add one of the following for a designer mustard: 3 tsp of crushed peppercorns, dill, oregano or basil, or ⅓ cup of mayonnaise.

Mint

Mint was originally used as a medicinal herb to treat stomach ache and chest pains. During the middle ages, powdered mint leaves were used to whiten teeth. Mint tea is a strong diuretic.

Menthol is an ingredient of many cosmetics and perfumes. Menthol and mint essential oils are also much used in medicine as component of many drugs, and are very popular in aromatherapy. A common use is as an anti-pruritic, especially in insect bite treatments.

Many ancient cultures appreciated the smell and aromatherapy properties of mint, from the ancient Hebrews, Greeks and Romans to the Japanese and the new frontier of the United States from aboard the Mayflower.

Mint's medicinal qualities are considered carminative, stimulative, stomachic, diaphoretic, and antispasmodic, as well as aiding in the relief of colds, flu and fevers, digestion, rheumatism, hiccups, stings, ear aches, motion sickness, flatulence and for throat and sinus ailments. There are also claims that a glass of creme de menthe helps with motion sickness.

Dill

Dill has long been cultivated as a herb throughout Europe and north Africa as well as in its native Asia. It was used by Egyptian doctors 5000 years ago and traces have been found in Roman ruins in Great Britain. In the Middle Ages it was thought to protect against witchcraft.

In Semitic languages it is known by the name of Shubit. The Talmud requires that tithes shall be paid on the seeds, leaves, and stem of dill. The Bible states that the Pharisees were in the habit of paying this tithe (Matthew 23:23); Jesus Christ is said to have rebuked them for tithing dill but omitting mercy.

The name Dill is thought to have originated from a Norse or Anglo-Saxon word 'dylle' meaning to soothe or lull, the plant having the carminative property of relieving gas.

Like caraway, its fern-like leaves are aromatic, and are used to flavour many foods, such as *gravad laks* (pickled salmon), borscht and other soups and pickles. The seeds are also used to flavour pickles. Dill is best when used fresh, as they lose their flavour rapidly if dried; however, freeze-dried dill leaves preserve their flavour relatively well for a few months. Even so, it is better to grow a supply of plants rather than store the leaves.

Dill oil can be extracted from the leaves, stems and seeds of the plant. As a sweet herb, Dill is not much used in this country. When used, it is for flavoring soups, sauces, etc., for which purpose the young leaves only are required. The leaves added to fish, or mixed with pickled cucumbers give them a spicy taste. Dill vinegar, however, forms a popular household condiment. It is made by soaking the seeds in vinegar for a few days before using.

The French use dill seeds for flavouring cakes and pastry, as well as for flavouring sauces.

Like the other umbelliferous fruits and volatile oils, both dill fruit and oil possess stimulant, aromatic, carminative and stomachic properties, making them of considerable medicinal value.

Oil of Dill is used in mixtures, or administered in doses of 5 drops on sugar, but its most common use is in the preparation of Dill Water, which is a common domestic remedy for the flatulence of infants, and is a useful vehicle for children's medicine generally.

To make herbal vinegar, a mild vinegar brand must be chosen, such as apple vinegar. Herbs, a clove of garlic and, if desired, a few pepper or allspice corns are then macerated for a couple of weeks. Many different herbs have been suggested, namely tarragon, thyme, bay leaves, chervil and bay leaves and chervil. Further optional herbs are rosemary, lemon balm, lovage, basil and even rue. Lemon-scented herbs (e.g., chameleon plant or lemon myrtle) are particularly effective. Perilla leaves can be used to give the vinegar both a subtle flavor and a most unusual colour. Dill adds depth and body to the product and should never be omitted. When ready, herbal vinegar may be used to prepare delicious sauces; most commonly, however, it is used for salads, which is delightful during winter when fresh herbs are sparse.

Drinking dill tea is recommended to overcome insomnia. A native to Europe, it is a Russian favourite and can be cultivated near the Arctic Circle. It was known as a medicinal herb to the ancient Greeks and Romans, where soldiers placed burned dill seeds on their wounds to promote healing. Medieval Europe could not grow it fast enough for love potions, casting spells and for protection against witchcraft. Carrying a bag of dried dill over the heart was considered protection against hexes.

"Therewith her Veruayne and her Dill, That hindreth Witches of their will" (Drayton, Nymphidia, 1627).

Caraway

Caraway is often recognized as the most typical spice of the German-speaking countries. It is an ancient spice of Central Europe. Caraway fruits have been found in Neolithic villages, and since Roman times there is lots of documentation for its numerous culinary and medicinal applications. Including a popular caraway-flavoured liquor, known as kummel in the USA, that is mostly produced and consumed in Northern Germany and Scandinavia.

Although caraway is a common plant of alpine meadows at low elevation, is was grown systematically in medieval monasteries, mainly to its extremely effective anti-flatulent powers.

Caraway is the spice that gives some European foods their characteristic flavor. Caraway's aroma does not harmonize with most other spices, except with garlic, yet popular with meat, roast pork, vegetables, sauerkraut, rye bread, potato dishes, pickle blends and some cheese varieties. Medicinally as a tisane for colic, and as a fragrance in soaps, lotions, and perfumes.

Caraway seeds are believed to have been used in Europe longer than any other condiment. Their use was first recorded in Egypt, in the medical papyrus of Thebes in 1552 B.C.

Anise

Anise is sweet and very aromatic, distinguished by its licorice-like flavor. It is used in a wide variety of regional and ethnic confections, including Greek stuffed vine leaves (*Dolma*), British Aniseed Balls, Australian Humbugs, New Zealand Aniseed Wheels, Italian *pizzelle*, German *pfeffernusse* and *springerle*, Netherland *Muisjes*, Norwegian *knotts*, and Peruvian *Picarones.* It is a key ingredient in Mexican *atole de anís* or *champurrado*, which is similar to hot chocolate, and taken as a digestive after meals in India.

It's believed to be one of the secret ingredients in the French liqueur Chartreuse. It is also used in some root beer such as Virgil's in the United States.

Some of its medicinal benefits include containing anethole, which is a phytoestrogen, being a mild anti-parasitic, and leaves that can treat digestive problems, toothaches, lice and scabies. Also considered to relieve menstrual cramps.

In aromatherapy, aniseed essential oil is used to treat colds and flu. Historically reputed to cure sleeplessness and scorpion stings, and known to freshen breath.

Very popular in Indian cuisine, with no distinction between anise and fennel, and used inter-changably. Great as a tea with a tablespoon of aniseed per cup, and even used as a heat sensor in the old locomotive train days, emitting a scent when machinery was overheating.

Cumin

Cumin has been in use since ancient times. Seeds, excavated at the Syrian site Tell ed-Der, have been dated to the second millennium BC. They have also been reported from several New Kingdom levels of ancient Egyptian archaeological sites.

Originally from Iran and Mediterranean region, cumin is mentioned in the Bible in both the Old Testament (Isaiah 28:27) and the New Testament (Matthew 23:23). The ancient Greeks kept cumin at the dining table, like we do with pepper today. Cumin became less popular in most of Europe during the Middle Ages, and was introduced to the Americas by Spanish colonists.

Superstition during the Middle Ages cited that cumin kept chickens and lovers from wandering. It was also believed that a happy life awaited the bride and groom who carried cumin seeds throughout the wedding ceremony.

Today, cumin is one of the most popular spices in the world, accompanying black pepper. Cumin seeds are used as a spice for their distinctive aroma, popular in Brazilian, Indian, African and Mexican cuisines. Cumin can also be found in Dutch cheeses like Leyden, in some traditional breads from France, and one of the spices in Chili Powder. Cumin is also added to curry dishes adding a warmness to stews and soups.

In folklore, medicinally, cumin tea (dry seeds boiled in hot water) is used to distinguish false labour (due to gas) from real labour, and to soothe acute stomach problems.

It's nutritional value consists of Vitamin A, B2, B3, B6, B9, B12, C, E, K, calcium, iron, magnesium, phosphorus, potassium, sodium and zinc.

Seaweed

Most people don't think of turning to the Earth's oceans for vegetables, yet there is a vast source of nutritious food available that is just now reaching the mainstream diet in the United States. Sea vegetables, or seaweed, are marine algae which is abundant all over the world. There are numerous forms of this seaweed, and they are among the most ancient life forms on earth. In many parts of the world, they have been harvested and eaten since long before land-based agriculture. Sometimes eaten fresh, but most often are dried, granulated and reconstituted, or boiled, granulated and added to other foods.

Sea vegetables are virtually fat-free, low calorie and one of the richest sources of minerals in any food. Because we, humans, started from the oceans, our blood contains many of the same minerals in very similar concentrations.

Seaweed can be made into a versatile, tasty gel that will set at room temperature. Its been used for centuries in the home as a mild laxative. Agar-agar is rich in iodine and trace elements, and used in jello-like products for vegetarians and vegans who prefer to avoid the horse-derived gelatin in foods.

These forgotten vegetables contain high amounts of calcium and phosphorous and are extremely high in magnesium, iron, iodine and sodium. For example, 1/4 cup of cooked hijiki contains over half the calcium that is found in a whole cup of milk and more iron than in an egg, making it perfect for vegans. It also contains vitamins A, B1, C and E, as well as protein and carbohydrates.

One of seaweed's most prominent health benefits is its ability to remove radioactive strontium and other heavy metals from our bodies. Whole brown seaweeds (not granulated) such as kelp contain alginic acid which binds with the toxins in the intestines rendering them indigestible and carries them out of the system.

The types of seaweed are:

Arame—A Japanese sea vegetable, with a mild flavor, Arame is dried and cut into thin strands, it can be added to soups or served as a vegetable side dish.

Hijiki—Found mostly in the Far East, containing the most calcium of any of the sea vegetables. In its natural state it is very tough; after harvesting it is dried, steamed and dried again. When cooked, it rehydrates and expands about five times its dry volume.

Kelp—This sea vegetable grows mainly in the north along the Pacific and Atlantic coastlines. The name kelp is European in origin and this plant is most often dried and sold whole, granulated or powdered. It can be sprinkled on foods like a salt, and a little goes a long way.

Kombu—can be used for soup stock or added to the bottom of a pot of rice or vegetables to help them keep from sticking; added to a pot of beans, Kombu helps them cook faster and renders them more digestible due to the high mineral content.

Wakame & Alaria—Although not originally found in the Celtic areas, these seaweeds are similar in characteristics. Wakame is a good source of protein, iron, calcium, sodium & other minerals and vitamins. Alaria is high in vitamin K and the B-vitamins as well as the minerals iodine and bromine.

Irish Moss—Irish Moss is most often used dried in relishes, breads, soups or fritters. Many people snack on this dried dulse straight out of the bag.

Nori—Probably our most culturally Celtic seaweed, now mainly cultivated as opposed to being obtained from the wild. In Ireland, it is known as *sloke* and in Scotland and Wales as *laver.* Gaelic people have long made flat breads from flour and nori, known as laver bread. Its most prominent use is as the wrapping for sushi, although it can be cut into strips, lightly toasted and used as a garnish as well. It is exceptionally high in vitamin A and protein. This is the type of seaweed that we will be using in our recipes.

Rosemary

Several studies done in the last a number of years show that oil from the leaves of this plant, sold as a spice for flavoring, can help prevent the development of cancerous tumors in laboratory animals. One study, at the UNB in New Jersey, showed that applying rosemary oil to the skin of animals reduced their risk of colon, lung or breast cancers in half.

Though these experiments have used rosemary oil to test the effectiveness in preventing cancer, the oil should not be taken internally. Even small doses can cause stomach, kidney and intestinal problems, and large amounts may be poisonous. Use a tea instead. Pregnant women should not use the herb medicinally (uteral cramping), although it's acceptable to use it as a seasoning.

Rosemary helps to relax muscles, the digestive tract and uterus muscles, yet when used in large amounts, the opposite occurs and causing internal irritation. Rosemary makes a pleasant-tasting tea. Use one teaspoon of crushed dried leaves in a cup of boiling water and steep for ten minutes.

For your skin, an infusion as a rinse can be used to lighten blond hair, as well as to condition and tone all hair. Consider rosemary as a natural toner and astringent and great for a refreshing bath.

Rosemary contains primarily borneol, camphor, eucalyptol and pinene in its essential oils, which can irritate the skin, yet be soothing when diluted in rheumatic liniments and ointments. Rosemary also contains chemicals called quinones, which have been shown in laboratory studies to inhibit carcinogens, making this herb ranked high on the list of cancer-prevention and reduction foods.

Salt

The story of sea salt began thousands of years ago, when the Celts discovered a way to harvest salt from the ocean using the sun, the wind, and shallow clay ponds. The ionizing action of the clay, combined with the salt workers skills, creates a salt harvest with quality mineral content, taste, texture, color and crystallization.

What studies have shown is a link between sodium and high blood pressure, yet this is when the salt that is used is mineral salt, and not natural sea salt. It is deemed that a balance of the sea salt minerals is necessary and more beneficial than eliminating sodium. The medical and scientific studies condemning table salt are justified, but for the fact that these studies examined refined white mineral salt, a biologically damaging, completely unnatural and chemicalized substance. In the industrial refining process, as many as 82 trace minerals and essential macro nutrients are forcibly removed, leaving only a single compound made of sodium and chlorine.

Your body uses mineral salts to create electrolytes. Electrolytes carry electrical currents throughout the body, sending messages and instructions to cells in all bodily systems. Electrolytes are also necessary for enzyme production, breaking down food, absorbing nutrients, muscle function, hormone production, a healthy immune function, proper regulation of bodily fluids, and adrenal health.

Real and natural sea salt can create a high-mineral soak that many have reported using successfully in the treatment of symptoms associated with arthritis & sore muscles. Finely ground sea salt makes a very effective nasal wash and gargle, helping to eliminate colds, allergies or sinus trouble symptoms.

True natural sea salt can come in a variety of colors. Sea salt gets it's color from the 100+ trace minerals missing from today's diet and is a healthier natural alternative to the overused table salt. Natural salt is dried from the sun and wind only and harvested by hand. Grey sea salt is about 84% sodium chloride, and the grey is from the contained important minerals.

Our bodies are created from the same elements of the earth and the oceans. Creatures living in natural salty ocean water would die in a mixture of table salt and water because it is chemically different from true salt. Our bodies are made up of water and salt in the right proportion with a mixture of minerals, all in balance. We need real natural sea salt in perfect balance to gain our health. Sea salt and natural spring water with all the trace minerals contained have that natural balance to get us to our optimum wellbeing.

Basically, table salt is harsh, having been mined, refined and bleached, with the minerals removed until it is virtually pure sodium chloride. Usually anti-caking chemicals and iodine are added. It is like a taste all to its own instead of enhancing the taste of the food.

Some of the names referring to natural sea salt are: real salt, natural salt, sea salt, grey salt, Himalayan salt, and Celtic salt. Yet read the label, as marketing can create a perception of natural when it isn't.

Pepper

Since the Middle Ages, pepper was the core of the European spice trade.

Pepper comes from several species of a vinous plant, the spice being the fruit, called peppercorns. Black pepper is the dried, unripe berry, about 1/8 inch in diameter. White pepper starts out the same as the black, but are allowed to ripen more fully on the vine. The outer shell is then removed by soaking the berries in water until the shell falls off, yielding a whiter, cleaner pepper. Green pepper is from the same fruit but is harvested before they mature. Pink pepper, which is not a vinous pepper, comes from the French island of Reunion. Pink peppercorns have a brittle, papery pink skin enclosing a hard, irregular seed, much smaller than the whole fruit.

On the pepper hot scale, black pepper is the hottest with an 8, white pepper with a 7, and green pepper with a 3.

Dried, ground pepper is one of the most common spices in European cuisine and its descendants, having been known and prized for both its flavour and its use as a medicine. The spiciness of black pepper is due to the chemical *piperine.* Ground black peppercorn, usually referred to simply as "pepper", may be found on nearly every dinner table in some parts of the world, often alongside table salt.

The word pepper is similar in many languages being *pippali* in Sanskrit, *piper* in Latin, *pipor* in the old English, *pfeffer* in German, *poivre* in French, and *peper* in Dutch. In the 16th century, pepper started referring to the unrelated New World chile peppers as well. The word pep is from the word pepper, regarding the spirit and energy of the spice.

Pepper, which in the early Middle Ages had been an item exclusively for the rich, started to become more of an everyday seasoning among those of more average means. Today, pepper accounts for one-fifth of the world's spice trade.

Thyme

The ancient Greeks used it in their baths and burnt it as incense in their temples, and it is believed that the spread of thyme throughout Europe was thanks to the Romans, to purify their rooms and to add aroma to cheeses and liqueurs.

It is a hardy potherb that can tolerate drought, take deep freezes and grow wild on mountain sides. For storing, this herb retains flavor better than other herbs, while flavoring strong but not overpowering.

Thyme is a good source of iron and is widely used in cooking meats, soups and stews. It has a particular culinary affect to lamb, tomatoes and eggs. Commonly sold in bunches of sprigs, a sprig being a single stem clipped from the plant. In your preparation of meals, use one third of the dried herb compared to the fresh herb, and add early in the cooking process as thyme takes it time to release its flavors.

Avoid thyme tea if pregnant as it has been used in some areas to cause uterine contractions in childbirth and possible placenta retaining.

Savory

Summer Savory (Satureja hortensis) is the better known of the Savory species. It is an annual, but otherwise is similar in use and flavor to the perennial Winter Savory.

Summer savory is a traditional popular herb on the east coast, where it is used in the same way sage is elsewhere. It is the main flavouring in dressing for stews, turkey and chicken. Dried, it is available year round in local grocery stores and unlike other herbs, you can add it to recipes in large generous heaping spoonfuls.

Summer savory is sweet and has a delicate aroma. It plays an important role in Bulgarian cuisine, where their tables will have three condiments: salt, paprika and savory. When these are mixed it is called *sharena sol* (colorful salt).

Winter savory is most often used as a culinary herb, but it also has marked medicinal benefits, especially upon the whole digestive system. This plant has a stronger action than the closely related summer savory.

Winter savory is reported to be a mild antiseptic, aromatic, carminative, digestive, mildly expectorant and stomachic. Taken internally, it is said to be a remedy for colic and a cure for flatulence, as well as to treat gastro-enteritis, cystitis, nausea, diarrhoea, bronchial congestion, sore throat and menstrual disorders, but it shouldn't be over consumed by pregnant women.

Continue to use your favorite herbs and spices and add some of the above mentioned ones. These aromatic additions can turn every meal into a flavorful and healthy one.

Vegetables

Traditional Celtic cuisine depends heavily on indigenous foodstuffs, such as root vegetables (potatoes, turnips, carrots), barley, oats, mutton and seafood such as haddock. Amongst farmers and the poor, meats such as mutton, chicken and beef would have been used sparingly. Common meals included soups such as Scotch Broth and Cock-a-leekie soup, using plenty of vegetables, and a meat stock but with small amounts of actual meat. Both of these dishes survive to this day.

In early history, many dishes would be seasoned simply with salt or pepper: porridge, made with oats, was traditionally flavored with salt, although sugar is more popular in modern times.

Because vegetable dish recipes were seldom mentioned in medieval cookbooks and historic writings, historians believed that vegetables were rarely eaten. We now know that vegetables were eaten daily and that the lack of notable mention was probably due to the vegetable's 'less important' food status.

Vegetables and herbs were found in abundance and an important food item in the diet of any traditional culture. Every continent has it's own plentiful and edible varieties, and the Celtic culture is no exception. It is assumed that scarce parchment shouldn't be wasted on writing down vegetable recipes. Some historic cookbooks actually point out that the ability to prepare vegetables is common knowledge and instructions unnecessary.

Onions are a good example of this attitude. This humble vegetable was a dietary staple yet considered peasant fare, for lower class meals, and not valued by the upper classes. In Chaucer's 'Summoner', his ill manners, ashen complexion and oily hair were blamed on onions and garlic. Even though the modest onion was given an undeserving snubbing, they were still eaten in great numbers, as nearly every garden grew onions and they are mentioned in historic cookbooks.

'Potherb' is the term in which virtually all plants were labeled. This included all vegetables, herbs, spices and even edible flowers. In a wide variety of historic writings including recipes, the word 'potherb' indicates some type of green.

'*Wortes*' was another common expression for certain vegetables, and included all leafy edible plants, such as parsley, but also included cabbage, spinach, and even onions & leeks.

Our modern salad differs slightly from medieval cookery. Many of the period cookbooks state vegetables to be served raw and with or without vinegar, oil, and salt. Salads, or '*salats*', were often served at the beginning of a meal as well.

The basic vegetables from the traditional Celtic diet will supply you with an amazing variety of nutritional factors in the form of vitamins, anti-oxidants, carbohydrates, fibre, healthy oils and minerals. The following is a list and description of the vegetables that were part of this healthy eating plan.

While you are adding significant amounts of the following amazing and almost forgotten vegetables, keep some of those contemporary favorites such as eggplant, zucchini, tomatoes, sweet potatoes, all shades of peppers, brocolli, some potatoes, and spinach. I would lessen or omit corn from your diet plan. In the old Celtic days, corn was considered cattle feed from the upper class, and the people that ate corn were considered lower class. But that is certainly not why we are avoiding it here. It is because, at last report, almost all corn was genetically altered and modified.

Garlic

Cultivated world wide. Garlic is related to onions, lilies, and shallots and mostly used as a seasoning or condiment. Allicin, is a powerful antibiotic and anti-fungal compound, as well as alliin, ajoene, enzymes, vitamin B, minerals and flavonoids, which are all found in garlic. It's health benefits include a lowering of cholesterol and triglycerides, and the inhibition of atherosclerosis. Aged Garlic extracts can improve the elastic properties of the aorta, lower blood homocysteine levels, and prevent some diabetic complications. It's diallyl sulphide properties make Garlic a cancer fighter, and can be used as a treatment for intestinal worms.

Garlic cloves continue to be used by health care experts as a remedy for chest infections, digestive disorders, and fungal infections. In such applications, garlic must be fresh and uncooked, or the allicin will be lost.

Garlic is mentioned in several Old English vocabularies of plants from the tenth to the fifteenth centuries, and is described by the herbalists of the sixteenth century.

Porrettes

Porrettes, also known as green onions, shallots, scallions and onions.

Green Onions. The common name scallion is associated with various members of the genus Allium, and one that lacks a fully-developed bulb. They are milder tasting than other onions and are typically used raw in salads in American cookery. Diced scallions are often used in soup, noodle dishes, seafood, and sauce in eastern cookery.

Scallions are also sometimes known as green onions in the U.S. and spring onions in England and Wales. In Australia they are known as eschallots, shallots, or spring onions. In Scotland, they are *cibies*. In the Republic of Ireland, *scallions*. The term green onion can also be used for immature specimens of the ordinary onion.

Onions appear to be somewhat effective against colds, heart disease, diabetes, osteoporosis, and other diseases and contain anti-inflammatory, anti-cholesterol, anti-cancer, and anti-oxidant components such as quercetin. Most historians agree that the onion has been cultivated for 5000 years or more. First by growing wild and being eaten, then grown domestically, at the same time, throughout the world. Onions would have been one of the earliest cultivated crops because they were less perishable, easily transportable, could be dried and preserved, easily grown, and in a variety of soils and climates.

By the Middle Ages, the three main vegetables of Celtic cuisine were beans, cabbage and onions. In addition to serving as a food for both the poor and the wealthy, onions were prescribed to alleviate headaches, snakebites and hair loss. They were also used as rent payments and wedding gifts.

Later, according to diaries of colonists, bulb onions were planted as soon as the settlers could clear the land in 1648. Onions have a variety of medicinal effects. Early American settlers used wild onions to treat colds, coughs, and asthma, and to repel insects. In Chinese medicine, onions have been used to treat angina, coughs, bacterial infections, and breathing problems. Today, the World Health Organization recognizes and supports the use of onions for certain treatments.

Onion extracts are rich in a variety of sulfides, provide some protection against tumor growth. In central Georgia where Vidalia onions are grown, mortality rates from stomach cancer are about one-half the average level for the United States. Studies in Greece have shown a high consumption of onions, garlic and other allium herbs to be protective against stomach cancer. Studies done in other countries show the same similar results.

When shopping, we tend to purchase the milder onion varieties, but studies show that these actually have less of the healthy benefits. To get the optimum benefits from onions, buy the stronger versions.

Leeks

Leeks are generally considered to have a finer flavor than the common onion. The edible portions are the white onion base and light green stalk. They are an essential ingredient of Cock-a-leekie and Vichyssoise soups, and can be used raw in salads.

The Ancient Egyptians, Greeks, and Romans, who distributed this vegetable across Europe, prized leeks. The Leek was the favorite vegetable of the Emperor Nero, who consumed it most often in soup form.

The leek is one of the national emblems of Wales, whose citizens wear it on St. David's Day. Even Shakespeare refers to the custom of wearing a leek as an ancient tradition in the play Henry V. The health benefits of leeks are almost exact to those of the onion.

Fennel

The word fennel developed from the Middle English *fenel* or *fenyl*, which came from the Old English *fenol* or *finol*, which in turn came from the Latin *feniculum* or *foeniculum*.

The bulb, foliage, and seeds of the fennel plant are widely used in many of the culinary traditions of the world. Fennel pollen is the most potent form of fennel, but also the most expensive. Dried fennel seed is an aromatic, anise-flavoured spice, brown or green in colour when fresh, slowly turning a dull grey as the seed ages. For cooking, green seeds are preferred. The leaves are delicately flavored and similar in shape to those of dill. The bulb is a crisp, hardy root vegetable and may be sauteed, stewed, braised, grilled, or eaten raw.

Fennel seeds are sometimes confused with those of anise, which are very similar in taste and appearance, though smaller. Fennel is also used as a flavouring in some natural toothpaste.

Fennel is popular in Mediterranean cuisine, both raw and cooked, in side dishes, salads, pastas, risotto, and vegetable dishes. Fennel seed is popular in Italian sausages and meatballs and in northern European rye breads.

The seeds do have a long medicinal history and are identified to have numerous uses, including to improve eyesight and to relieve jaundice. As early as the Third Century, Hippocrates prescribed fennel to combat infant colic. Today fennel is known for relieving gastrointestinal disorders, indigestion, spasms in the digestive system, act as a diuretic, a pain reliever and fever-reducer.

Watercress

Watercress is the richest natural source of a compound called phenylethylisothiocyanate, or PEITC1, which gives the plant its unique peppery flavor. Over 50 scientific studies have proven that PEITC is not just a potent inhibitor of cancer development, but that it has the ability to kill cancer cells and prevent cancer-causing agents being metabolized into carcinogens, as well to stimulate enzymatic activity involved in the detoxification of carcinogens.

In 2000, a study revealed that watercress also contained another glucosinolate, called methylsulphinylalkyl glucosinolate, a precursor of a range of methylsulphinylalkyl isothiocyanates (MEITC) usually found in broccoli and brussel sprouts, and that together these compounds formed a more potent anti-cancer weapon.

Watercress is a fast-growing, aquatic or semi-aquatic, perennial originating from Europe to central Asia and one of the oldest known leaf vegetables. These plants are members of the cabbage (Brassica) family, botanically related to garden cress and mustard, all of which are noted for a peppery, tangy flavor. Watercress contains significant amounts of iron, calcium and folic acid, in addition to vitamins A & C.

Rue

Or Rew, is a hardy, evergreen, somewhat shrubby plant, and a native of Southern Europe. The stem is woody in the lower part, the leaves are bluish-green, and are known to emit a powerful, disagreeable odor and have an exceedingly bitter, acrid and nauseous taste. Rew was generally used to add flavoring to most foods, and can best be used heated to release the oils, then discard the leaves. Because of its bitter strength, Rue isn't as popular with today's cooks.

Purslane

Or Puerslayn, also known as Pigweed, Little Hogweed or Pusley, is an annual succulent from the Portulacaceae family. Although purslane is considered a weed in the United States, it can be eaten as a leaf vegetable. It has a slightly sour and salty taste and is used fresh as a salad, or cooked like spinach. Due to its mucilaginous quality it is also great for soups and stews.

Purslane contains more Omega-3 fatty acids than any other leafy vegetable plant. It also contains vitamins C and B, as well as dietary minerals, such as magnesium, calcium, potassium and iron. Also present are two types of anti-multi mutagenics that are contained in the reddish and yellowish pigments.

Dandelions

Dandelions are native to temperate areas of the Northern Hemisphere of the Old World. While the dandelion is considered a weed by many gardeners, the plant does have several culinary and medicinal uses. The plant can be eaten cooked or raw in various forms, such as in soup or salad. They are probably closest in character to mustard greens. Usually the young leaves and unopened buds are eaten raw in salads, while older leaves are cooked. Raw leaves have a slightly bitter taste. Dandelion salad is often accompanied with hard boiled eggs.

Dandelion flowers can be used to make dandelion wine or a dandelion flower jam, usually containing citrus fruits. The leaves are high in vitamin A, vitamin C and iron. Ground roasted dandelion root can be used as a coffee substitute. Drank before meals, it is believed to stimulate digestive functions. Sold in most health food stores, often in a mixture, it is considered an excellent cleansing tonic for the liver.

Dandelion root is a registered drug in Canada, sold as a diuretic. A leaf decoction can be drunk to "purify the blood", for the treatment of anemia, jaundice, and also for nervousness. "Dandelion and Burdock" is a soft drink that has long been popular in the United Kingdom.

Used as medicinal and edible, the Dandelion is very nutritious, having more vitamins and minerals than most vegetables. An infusion of the root encourages the steady elimination of toxins from the body.

The trace minerals are just part of a package of some 64 nutrients and health-promoting substances which have been found in dandelions by plant chemists around the world.

But Dandelions are bitter, yet easy to mask it by serving the dandelions with breads and pastas, tomato-based sauces, sweet dressings, cheese, meats and condiments such as vinegar, lemon and garlic. Properly prepared, everyone now can enjoy the flavor as well as the nutritional benefits of dandelions. You can also add dried dandelions to your tea blend.

Collect dandelion leaves in the spring before the flower buds appear or they are too bitter to eat. Most importantly, collect these greens from area that have not been sprayed with herbicides or pesticides. Avoid well travelled roads where spraying as well as the metals and toxins from vehicle exhausts have all landed on nearby plants.

Sorrel

The common sorrel, or spinach dock, is a perennial herb, which grows plentifully in meadows in most parts of Europe and has been cultivated as a leaf vegetable for centuries. The edible leaves have a flavor that is very similar to that of Kiwifruit or sour wild strawberries. The leaves may be added to salads to sharpen the taste and often puréed in soups and sauces. The plant contains oxalic acid, which contributes to its characteristic flavor, but should be avoided by people with rheumatic-type complaints, kidney or bladder stones.

The spring leaves flavor is mildest, and it is used in salads and cooked as a vegetable. A few slivered young sorrel leaves add a refreshing touch to any sandwich. The fresh young leaves can be combined with other herbs in salads, or cooked and served like spinach, usually in combination with either Swiss chard or spinach.

Cream of sorrel soup is a famous Old World dish, and salmon with sorrel sauce is a popular dish in France. The First Nations of Canada and the United States have used this plant, also known as sour grass or sour weed, as a food and medicine. Sheep sorrel is a popular ingredient of many folk remedies and the tea was used traditionally as a diuretic and to treat fevers, inflammation and scurvy. Sheep sorrel was considered the most active herb in Essiac for stimulating cellular regeneration, detoxification and cleansing, based on reports by Rene Caisse and her doctor colleague who did studies with mice bearing abnormal growths on the original eight herb formula.

Sheep sorrel contains: rutin, flavone glycosides, hyperin, vitamins C, A, B complex, D, E, K, P, U, calcium, phosphorus, magnesium, potassium, iron, sulphur, copper, iodine, manganese, zinc, carotenoids, chlorophyll, organic acids (malic, oxalic, tannic, tartaric and citric), phytoestrogens, anthraquinones, aloe emodin, chrysophanol, rhein, and physcion. As great as sorrel is, use on a limited daily basis as it works very well as a laxative.

Mustard Greens

Mustard greens are the leaves of the mustard plant, Brassica juncea. The leaves of mustard greens can have either a crumpled or flat texture and may have either toothed, scalloped, frilled or lacey edges. Besides the nutritious greens, this plant also produces the brown seeds that are used to make Dijon mustard. Mustard greens, also known as green mustard cabbage and the Indian mustard plant, are considered to be an essential element in soul food. These are more pungent than the closely related greens of kale, cabbage, and collard greens, and are very frequently mixed with these milder greens in a dish of "mixed greens", which can also often include wild greens such as dandelion.

Mustard greens are also extremely high in Vitamin A and Vitamin K among other important nutrients, including 6 more vitamins, 7 minerals, dietary fiber protein, and health-promoting phytochemicals known as glucosinolates.

These greens are considered serious free radical scavengers, working against conditions such as asthma, heart disease, cancer prevention, arthritis and menopausal symptoms. Those with thyroid conditions should avoid mustard greens as one of it components can interfere with its functioning.

Kale

Kale is a form of cabbage, and another vegetable that belongs to the Brassica family. It is highly nutritious, has powerful antioxidants, and offers many health benefits.

Kale is rich in vitamin K. One cup, boiled, has 1062.10 mcg of Vitamin K, which is 10 times the daily value. And should be avoided by those who take anti-coagulants, like warfarin. Other important components are vitamin A, vitamin C, vitamin B6, riboflavin, thiamine, niacin, folate, manganese, calcium, potassium, iron, magnesium, protein, dietary fiber, and omega 3 fatty acids.

Because of Kale's brassica family connection, it is considered to have anti-cancer properties, able to reduce the development of cataracts and macular degeneration of the eyes, remove toxins from the body, improve the immune system, promote and maintain weight loss, prevention of constipation, atherosclerosis and high blood pressure.

Kale is a great source of non-dairy calcium, low in calories at 36 calories per cup, free of saturated fats, and is *not* a highly allergenic food.

Cabbage

The health benefits of cabbage are being recognized and proven weekly. This includes the treatment of constipation, stomach ulcers, headache, excess weight, eczema, jaundice, scurvy, rheumatism, arthritis, gout, eye disorders, heart diseases, ageing, detoxifying tissues, rheumatism, arthritis, renal calculi, skin conditions, improving the immune system, infection and colds, depression, intestinal disorders, and Alzheimer's disease.

Yet it is one of the least expensive vegetables available, as well as be quite versatile. It is widely used throughout the world, eaten cooked or raw as salad and is a very popular vegetable.

Although it is not a citrus, cabbage is abundant in Sulphur and Vitamin C.

Iodine, also naturally found in cabbage, helps with the proper performance of the brain and the nervous system, as well as Vitamin E for the care of skin, eyes and hair.

In order to get that cabbage in you, discover how it can be prepared that makes it more interesting to you. Coleslaw is liked by many, but preferred when it is grated and not sliced and diced. Like pickled foods?, then sauerkraut is for you, a great addition to any lunch or dinner. You can also juice cabbage and mix it with other fruits and vegetables. Sauté shredded cabbage and top with spaghetti sauce for a carb-free and white-flour-free spaghetti. Try the Cabbage Roll Soup recipe in the Vegetable Recipe Section.

Beets

The health benefits of beets include anemia, digestion, constipation, piles, blood circulation, kidney disorders, skin care, dandruff, gall bladder disorders, cancer, and heart diseases.

Beets or beetroots, belong to the Chenopodiaceous family. Health benefits of beet roots can be attributed to their richness in nutrients, vitamins and minerals. They are a source of carotenoids and lutein/zeaxanthin. Beets are also rich in dietary fiber, vitamin C, magnesium, iron, copper and phosphorus. Beets are a source of beneficial flavonoids called anthycyanins. They are very low in calories but have the highest sugar content of all vegetables. They are also used to make refined sugar.

Beetroot is also added as an ingredient to salads, soups and pickles and also used as a natural coloring agent. Even though beets are available throughout the year they are still considered seasonal vegetables.

The roots and leaves of beets have plenty of medicinal and healthy benefits and uses, like:

- the fiber and the betaine helps to reduce cholesterol and triglycerides and therefore lowering the risk for heart related problems, as well as stimulating the function of the liver;

- the B vitamin folate helps the healthy development of babies' in vitro;

- the pigment betacyaninis contains anti-cancer components reducing the risk of cell mutations and slowing down tumor growth;

- Vitamin C and natural beta-carotene to prevent asthma symptoms and prevent lung cancer;

- complex carbohydrates for natural energy;

- Vitamin A, or beta-carotene to prevent cataracts and macular degeneration;

- flavonoids and vitamin C to support capillaries structure;

- potassium to lower the risk of stroke;

- boron to produce healthy hormone levels;

- known to cure fevers and constipation and other digestive disorders;

- beet leaves good for curing wounds.

Beets, and the previously mentioned Sorrel, both contain oxalates, which when consumed in excess, could aggravate, diagnosed or undiagnosed, kidney or gallbladder problems.

Wild Celery

It was wild celery back in the early days, now all celery is farm grown and found in our grocers produce section. Besides celery consisting of great amounts of water, water that we need to add every day, the health benefits of this quiet salad vegetable are surprising.

These rich nutrients are vitamin C, amino acids, boron, calcium, chlorine, essential fatty acids, folate, inosital, iron, magnesium, manganese, phosphorous, potassium, selenium, sulfur, zinc, fiber, vitamin A, vitamin B1, B2, B3, B5, B6, C, E, and K.

The health benefits of celery include the following: reducing blood pressure, reducing cholesterol, anti-septic properties for bladders conditions, anti-inflammatory properties against arthritis, rheumatism and gout, reducing swelling and pain around joints, the anti-cancer components of phthalides and ployacetylenes, improving immune systems, reducing cold symptoms and the severity of asthma, preventing free radical damage, reducing inflammatory conditions, regulating fluid balances, can relieve migraines, and aids in relieving ophthalmologic conditions.

Celery also has a high calcium content and can help to calm nerves. All parts of the celery can be eaten, including the seed, root and leaves. Drinking celery juice before meals will also help reduce weight. But avoid celery seeds if you are pregnant, as these may cause the uterus to contract.

Turnip

The turnip, also known as Rutabaga, was a prized vegetable in that it could be left in the ground until the next harvest, thus preventing a total famine for the Celts.

Turnip is a root vegetable, which is easy to grow, and not too fussy about its soil conditions. The greens are similar to mustard greens in their flavor and nutrition. Turnips are an excellent source of potassium, sodium, magnesium, phosphorus, iron, zinc, copper, manganese, selenium and calcium.

Turnips are also rich in Vitamin C, contain a good amount of choline and small amounts of Vitamin K, B6, thiamin, niacin, folate and Pantothenic acid. And only about 70 calories per cup.

Again, another vegetable from the Brassica family. These health benefits include treating arthritis, lowering the risk of obesity, high blood pressure, diabetes, and cancers of the stomach, pancreas, bladder and lung diseases. Turnips help prevent cataracts and cardiovascular disease.

Radish

Famous for being a salad vegetable, the Radish, is a root crop, pungent or sweet in taste with a lot of juice. Radishes can be white, red, purple or black, long cylindrical or round in shape. They are eaten raw, cooked or pickled. The oil obtained from the seeds of radish is also used. The other parts of radish which are consumed are the leaves, the flowers, the pods and the seeds. The scientific name of radish is Raphanus Sativus which belongs to the Brassicaceae family. The benefits of radish against certain ailments and on certain body parts are jaundice, reducing hemorrhoids, urinary disorders, aiding in weight loss, anti-cancer properties, the special anti-cancer properties against leucoderma, skin disorders, kidney disorders, insect bites, fever, respiratory disorders, bronchitis, asthma, allergies, liver and gallbladder, circulation, and dyspepsia.

Nettle

Nettle, also known as stinging nettle, has been used for centuries to treat allergy symptoms, particularly hay fever which is the most common allergy problem. It contains biologically active compounds that reduce inflammation. Dr. Andrew Wiel, M.D., author of Natural

Health/Natural Medicine, says he knows of nothing more effective than nettle for allergy relief. And his statement is backed up by studies at the National College of Naturopathic Medicine in Portland, Oregon.

Decongestants, antihistamines, allergy shots and even prescription medications such as Allegra and Claritin treat only the symptoms of allergies and tend to lose effectiveness over a period of time. They can also cause drowsiness, dry sinuses, insomnia and high blood pressure. Nettle has none of these side effects. It can be used on a regular basis and has an impressive number of other benefits most notably as a treatment for prostate enlargement.

It's properties are an incredible reading list, being that it is an analgesic, anti-inflammatory, anti-allergenic, anti-anaphylactic, anti-rheumatic, anti-asthmatic, anti-convulsant, anti-dandruff, anti-histamine, astringent, decongestant, depurative, diuretic, haemostatic, hypoglycaemic, hypotensive, galactagogue, immunomodulator, prostate tonic, and a stimulating tonic.

Which all means in could be used for seasonal allergies, arthritis, bronchitis, bursitis, gingivitis, laryngitis, prostatitis, rhinitis, sinusitis, tendinitis, BPH, rheumatism and other inflammatory conditions, high blood pressure, hair loss, anemia, excessive menstruation, hemorrhoids, eczema, gout, neuralgia, Alzheimer's disease, asthma, bladder infections, hives, kidney stones, multiple sclerosis, PMS, prostate enlargement and sciatica. Consider adding nettle leaves to your next cup of tea to gain some of these benefits.

Parsnips

Parsnips, or welsh carrots, are often overlooked when it comes to juicing and they really shouldn't be. Make sure to make the most of this winter vegetable when it is in season. Parsnip juice is a sweet juice similar to carrot juice but has its own distinctive taste. By itself the sweetness of parsnip juice can be a bit full on so try mixing it with other juices such as apples, spinach and celery.

When selecting parsnips for juicing look for produce that is cream in colour, firm to the touch and of good weight. Avoid parsnips that have been left in the ground for too long as their fibres become woody rather than succulent.

If your parsnips are organic then simply remove any attached soil, rinse the parsnips and remove the top and the tail. Cut the parsnip into small pieces that are suitable for feeding into your juicers feeding chamber. If your parsnips are not organic then you may want to peel them first as you would carrots.

The health benefits of parsnips are again under-rated. Parsnip juice contains far less calories than carrot juice and so is a valuable ingredient in juice recipes that aim to help weight loss. Parsnips are a good source of folic acid, potassium, sulphur and vitamin C. This makes parsnip juice a valuable ally in the quest for healthy skin. Parsnip has been associated with improving bronchial tube functioning in the lungs and so may be of benefit to those who suffer from asthma.

Peas

In early times, peas were grown mostly for their dry seeds. In modern times, however, peas are usually boiled or steamed, which breaks down the cell walls and makes the taste sweeter and the nutrients more bio-available. Along with broad beans and lentils, these formed an important part of the diet of most people in Europe during the Middle Ages.

By the 1600s and 1700s, it had become popular to eat peas green, meaning raw. In France and England, the eating of green peas was said to be "both a fashion and a madness". New varieties of peas were developed during this time which became known as garden peas and English peas. Later, the popularity of green peas spread to the United States where Thomas Jefferson grew more than 30 types of peas on his estate. With the modern invention of canning and freezing of foods, green peas became available year-round, and not just in the spring.

Fresh peas are often eaten boiled and flavored with butter and/ or spearmint as a side dish vegetable. Salt and pepper are also commonly added to peas when served. Fresh peas are also used in pot pies, salads and casseroles. Pod peas, sugar peas, or the flatter snow peas, are used in stir-fried dishes.

In India, fresh peas are used in various dishes such as *aloo matar* (curried potatoes with peas) or *matar paneer* (paneer cheese with peas), though they can be substituted with frozen peas as well.

Dried peas are often made into a soup or simply eaten on their own. In many Asian countries, the peas are roasted and salted, and eaten as snacks. In the UK, dried yellow split peas are used to make pease pudding, also known as pease porridge, a traditional dish. In North America, a similarly traditional dish is split pea soup.

Pea soup is eaten in many other parts of the world, in Sweden it is called *ärtsoppa*, and is eaten as a traditional Swedish food which predates the Viking era. This food was made from a fast-growing pea that would mature in a short growing season. *Ärtsoppa* was especially popular among the many poor who traditionally only had one pot and everything was cooked together for a dinner using a tripod to hold the pot over the fire.

In the United Kingdom, dried, rehydrated and mashed marrowfat peas, known by the public as mushy peas, are popular, especially when served with fish and chips or meat pies. Sodium bicarbonate is sometimes added to soften the peas. In 2005, a poll of 2,000 people revealed the pea to be the UK's 7th favorite culinary vegetable.

The nutritional value of peas are Vitamin A, beta-carotene, lutein, zeaxanthin, thiamine (B1), Riboflavin (B2), Niacin (B3), Pantothenic acid (B5), Vitamin B6, Folate (B9), Vitamin C, Calcium, Iron, Magnesium, Phosphorus, Potassium, and Zinc.

Potatoes

The potato was introduced into Ireland in the second half of the 17th century, initially as a garden crop. It eventually came to be the main food crop of the poor. As a food source, the potato is extremely valuable in terms of the amount of energy produced per unit area of crop. The potato is also a good source of many vitamins and minerals, particularly vitamin C (especially when fresh).

Potatoes were cultivated by much of the population at a next-to-survival level and the diet of this period consisted mainly of potatoes supplemented with buttermilk. Potatoes were also used as a food for pigs that were fattened-up for cold winter months.

The reliance on potatoes as a staple crop meant that the people of Ireland were vulnerable to poor potato harvests. Consequently several famines occurred throughout the 17th and 18th centuries. The first great famine of 1739 was the result of extreme cold weather but the famine of 1846 to 1849 was caused by potato blight which easily spread throughout the Irish crop which heavily dependent on a single variety, the Lumper.

Vegetable Recipes

Generally, the vegetables that were popular back then were the vegetables that could keep without refrigeration. Any of the vegetables mentioned in this diet are all vegetables you could juice as well, and get the added benefits of juicing. Consider raw versions of your vegetables, in order to obtain the enzymes that are found in only raw fruits and vegetables. Vegetables are the most important part of any health program or weight loss plan.

Some of these cultural recipes call for what may be considered sizeable amounts of oils and butters. In order the get the benefits while keeping down the calorie count, consider frying in Coconut Oil, with some water. Nowadays, corporations are making some products natural enough for most of us to consider using. There are some cooking sprays available with ingredient lists that read: Extra Virgin Olive Oil, Water, Emulsifier (being Soya Lecithin and Alcohol), and Vitamin E as a preservative. Decide which method is best for you. Perhaps a combination of techniques, such as frying with a spray or a Coconut Oil/water blend, and save the butters for other recipes.

Earlier in this chapter, the benefits of these main vegetables are listed, and one important common denominator with a lot of these vegetables are that they belong to the Brassica (or Brassicaceae) family of vegetables. A vegetable family that our bodies are desperately missing and much needing.

Colcannon

6 medium potatoes, peeled and quartered

4 cups shredded cabbage (some use kale)

¼ cup butter

about 1 cup milk

6 green onions, diced

Salt and Pepper to taste

Boil the peeled quartered potatoes in lightly salted water until mashable while shredding and boiling the cabbage in a pot, 5-8 minutes. Drain cabbage, add half of the butter and all green onion and return to heat. When potatoes are done, drain well. Add up to 1 cup of milk and mash to a smooth consistently, usually thinner than regular mashed potatoes. Add the rest of the butter, cabbage mixture and season with salt and pepper.

Glazed and Baked Turnips

5 medium turnips, peel and slice about 1/4 inch thick

1 beef bouillon cube in the pot water, or broth

1/4 cup melted butter

2 T brown sugar

Black or red crushed pepper to taste

Salt to taste

Cook turnips until tender then drain and place in casserole dish. Drizzle with melted butter, sprinkle with sugar and pepper. Place in 350 degree oven for about 15 minutes until flavors are blended. Serve hot. Serves 4.

Leek and Sausage Soup

1 large onion

fresh black pepper

2 T cooking oil

2 leeks

16 oz of cream, (use less or use whole milk)

16-20 oz chicken and/or vegetable stock

1 T sage

3 bay leaves

juice of one lemon

eight sausages (or less)

Cook sausages and sauté onions and washed thinly sliced leeks on low heat. Cook all till golden. Slice sausages and add to leek and onion mixture, the add the broth and additional water as needed. Add the cream, lemon juice and bay leaves and simmer on low heat.

Stir-fried Cabbage

1 medium head cabbage (about 2 lbs.)

2 medium sized carrots

1 green pepper

2 T vegetable oil

1 tsp salt

Soy sauce (optional)

1/4 tsp garlic powder

1/2 tsp sugar

1/4 cup broth or water

1/2 tsp oriental sesame oil

Coarsely shred cabbage, cut carrots in match stick pieces, and cut pepper into 3/4 inch pieces and set aside. Heat oil in a skillet over medium-high and add salt and garlic; stir-frying for a short 5-10 seconds. Quickly add the cabbage, carrots and pepper; stir-fry 10 seconds. Lower heat, add sugar and broth. Cover and steam for 2 to 5 minutes. Add soy sauce at serving if desired. Makes 6 servings. But because this particular recipe is really low in fats and calories, and high in nutrients, eat as much as you like.

Beet Salad and Walnut Dressing

2/3 lb fresh beets

4 tsp red wine vinegar

3/4 tsp sea salt

1/4 tsp pepper

4 T oil

1/4 cup broken walnut pieces

Salad greens

Peel and grate beets. Shake salt, pepper, and vinegar in jar until salt dissolves then add oil and shake again until blended. Toss beets with dressing and nuts and serve with salad greens.

Cream of Celery Soup

1 onion, minced

1-2 cups celery leaves and stalks

1 bay leaf

4 sprigs parsley

1 sprig thyme

1 whole clove

1 cup cold water

1 tsp salt

1 T flour

1 T butter (room temperature)

16 oz milk, scalded (use less or dilute with water)

salt, pepper, nutmeg, to taste

1 egg yolk, well beaten

2 cups light cream, (could lessen and dilute with water)

fresh parsley and paprika (for garnishing)

In a medium saucepan, combine the onion and finely diced celery with 1 cup cold water and 1/2 teaspoon salt. Tie together (using cotton kitchen string or tea leaf holder) the bay leaf, parsley, thyme and clove and toss in. Simmer over medium-low heat for 30-35 minutes.

Cream together butter and flour and in a small saucepan scald the milk. Stir the butter and flour mixture into the hot milk. Then add this to the onion/celery/water saucepan and simmer on low for 15 minutes. Remove package of herbs and discard.

To make this the perfect creamy soup, process the soup in a food processor or blender until smooth. Return to saucepan, add the light cream, heat, add a beaten egg yolk and mix well. Season and serve.

Celery and Parsnip Stew

1/2 lb parsnips

2 medium onions, chopped

3/4 lb celery, chopped

2 T butter

1 T flour

1 cup stock or water

2 tsp dried parsley

1 bay leaf

1/2 to 3/4 tsp thyme

Freshly ground pepper to taste

Peel the parsnips and chop into 1/2 to 1 inch pieces. Melt the butter in a large saucepan; add the onions and celery, sautéing until golden but not browned. Mix in the flour, let cook for 2 minutes, and add parsnips, stock, bouillon or water, parsley, bay leaf and thyme. Stir, cover and cook over medium-low heat, stirring frequently. Cook for 10 to 15 minutes or until tender. Remove the bay leaf, season with pepper to taste and serve.

Chilled Carrot and Ginger Soup

3 T butter, or a few of splashes of olive oil (or half of each)

pinch of salt

1 pound carrots, chopped

1 medium onion, chopped

1 stalk of celery, peeled and chopped

1 teaspoon ginger, chopped or grated

5 cups broth or stock

Zest of half a lime

Juice of one lime

Heat butter or oil in soup pot on medium low, and add onions, carrots, celery and salt. Sauté until onions and carrot are soft. Add ginger and cook for a minute or two more. Add broth, cook for 5 to ten minutes at a low boil. To puree the soup, use a blender or food processor. Add the lime zest and juice, and chill and serve.

Borscht Soup

Usually a vegetarian soup, although you could add a little meat. Borscht is famous throughout Europe and every country has its own special version.

Oil or butter to sauté in

1 large onion, chopped

12 cups stock or broth

6 large beets, peeled and roughly chopped

1 28 ounce can of diced tomatoes

Juice of 1 lime

Salt and pepper to taste

Sour cream, chopped green onions for garnish

Heat oil or butter in soup pot on medium low heat. Add onions and salt, sauté until onions are soft. Add remaining ingredients except garnish. Bring to a boil, reduce and cook covered for about an hour. For a creamier texture, use a blender to puree. When serving, top with a dollop of sour cream and a sprinkle of diced green onion or chives.

Onion Soup

4 large sweet white onions, sliced about 1/4 inch thick

3-6 cloves of garlic, chopped finely

Olive oil, to sauté in

Butter (optional)

1 Bay Leaf

A few sprigs of fresh thyme

Salt and pepper to taste

1 T of Dijon mustard

8 cups stock or broth

1/8 cup finely cut oatmeal

Heat olive oil and butter in soup pot on medium low heat and add onions, garlic, salt, pepper, bay leaf and thyme. Sauté onions till golden brown, approx 30 minutes, or until done, and on low heat.

Remove the bay leaf and thyme sprigs, add the mustard, stock, oatmeal and stir. Bring to a boil and reduce heat to simmer for 15 minutes.

Roasted Garlic Soup

8 cups water

2 or 3 bulbs of Garlic

1 cup Barley or Oatmeal

2-4 T Dill

2 T Parsley

1/4 tsp, to start with, Jalapeños, or jarred crushed red pepper

1/8 tsp coarse Black Pepper

2 medium diced or grated carrots

2 diced celery stalks

1/2 cup of finely chopped oatmeal

juice of one lemons, or 2 T

Boil water and preheat oven for roasting the garlic. When oven is ready, place on a roaster pan and roast in oven for approx 10 minutes. Start adding your herbs and vegetables to the boiling water, and when garlic is ready, peel and put in soup. Add Jalapenos, and when soup is ready, add the lemon juice. Simmer for 30 minutes.

Cabbage Roll Soup

1/2 head of cabbage, chopped

1 14.5 oz tin of stewed diced tomatoes

1 carrot, diced

1 medium onion, diced

1 celery stalk, diced

2 cloves garlic, chopped finely

Olive oil for sautéing

8 cups stock or broth

1/2 cup oatmeal, any size

Salt and pepper to taste

Heat oil in soup pot, add the onion, celery and carrot and a bit of salt. Cook on medium-low heat for about 5 minutes. Add the garlic and cook for two or three minutes more. Add remaining ingredients. Bring to a boil, reduce heat and simmer for 20 to 30 minutes, depending on how coarsely the cabbage was chopped. The cabbage should wilt, and then cook for about 10 minutes more to allow flavors to mix.

Cock-a-Leekie Soup

Approximately 1 pound of chicken or less, roasted chicken leftovers would be perfect

12 leeks cleaned and roughly chopped

8 cups chicken stock or water

1/4 cup of oatmeal or barley

4-6 cooked diced pitted prunes

1 tsp brown sugar

Salt and pepper to taste Parsley and thyme to taste

2 or 3 bay leaves

Put the chicken and leeks in the soup pot and cover with cold water or stock. Bring to a gentle boil. Add the salt, pepper, bay leaves, parsley allow to simmer for at least two hours. Add the oats or barley to the soup, plus the prunes, and simmer for another 30 minutes.

Wilted Coleslaw

1 head green cabbage, cored and sliced thin

2 carrots, peeled and grated

1 medium white onion, diced

For the Dressing:

1 cup white wine vinegar

3/4 cup canola oil

1/2 cup honey

1 T lemon juice

2 T mustard seeds

1 T salt

1/2 tsp freshly ground black pepper

In a large, non-aluminium mixing bowl, combine the cabbage, carrots and onion.

For the dressing, in a non-aluminium saucepan over medium heat, mix the vinegar, oil, honey, lemon juice, mustard seeds, salt, and pepper. Bring to a boil, stirring often. Take the dressing off the heat; immediately pour it over the vegetables. Toss well, cover, and refrigerate for at least 6 hours before serving.

For a cold version of the great Coleslaw recipe, make your dressing then put it in the fridge to cool. Just before serving, add the cooled dressing and toss.

Buttered Spinach Wortes

18 oz spinach, very finely chopped

18 oz mustard greens, leave and stems, very finely chopped

(or a combinations of greens)

5 T coarsely chopped garlic

4-6 fresh hot green chillies

1½-2 tsp salt

5-6 T cornmeal flour

3 T ghee or vegetable oil

1 medium-large onion, 4oz, finely chopped

2 inch piece of fresh ginger, peeled and cut into thin long slivers

2 medium-sized tomatoes, finely chopped

a generous dollop of unsalted butter

Combine the spinach, mustard greens, garlic, chillies, salt and 24 oz water in a large saucepan. Cook on high heat, bring to a boil, then cover, and simmer gently for 1¾ hours or until the stems of the mustard greens have turned buttery soft. While on simmer, add 5 T of the cornmeal flour, stirring with a whisk or green masher. After blending in the cornmeal, mash the greens until they are smooth. The greens will thicken but if a little watery, add another T or two of cornmeal.

Heat the ghee or oil in a separate pan over medium-high heat. Add the onion, sauté till golden-brown, add ginger, continue till mixture is medium-brown. Add tomatoes and continue till the tomatoes have softened and browned a little. Then pour this mixture over the greens and stir it in. Empty the greens into a serving dish, top with a dollop of butter and serve.

From a Fifteenth Century Cookbook:

Buttered Wortes. Take al manor of good herbes that thou may gete, and do bi ham as is forsaid; putte hem on the fire with faire water; put ther-to clarefied buttur a grete quantite. Whan thei ben boyled ynough, salt hem; late none otemele come ther-in. Dise brede small in disshes, and powre on the wortes, and serue hem forth.

Buttered Wortes (translated):

8 cups of any combination of spinach, cabbage, beet greens, onion, leeks, parsley, etc., chopped

1/2 stick (1/8 lb.) of butter

salt to taste

1 cup unseasoned croutons

Cover greens with water; add butter and bring to a boil; add salt. Reduce heat & cook until tender; drain. Place croutons in serving bowl and cover with cooked greens.

A Herb and Flower Salad recipe from 1390 AD Scotland:

Salat: "Take persel (parsley), sawge, grene garlec, chibolles, (spring onions), oynouns, leek, borage, myntes, porrettes (a type of leek), fennel, and town cressis, rew, rosemaye, purslayne; lave and wasche hem clene. Pike hem. Pluk hem small with thyme hande, and mingle hem wel with rawe oile; lay on vynegar and salt, and serve it forth."

Herb and Flower Salad, a translated and contemporary version:

2 cups watercress

1 bunch mustard greens

2 oz fresh parsley sprigs

1 leek; finely sliced

6 green onions; chopped

1 fennel bulb; sliced into match sticks

Dressing:

Red sage leaves

Mint leaves

1 fresh rosemary sprig chopped

1 clove garlic

1 T wine vinegar

salt & pepper to taste

6 T olive oil

Add together the greens in a large bowl, which has been rubbed well with a garlic clove. Place the wine vinegar, seasonings and olive oil into a screw-topped jar and shake well to blend. Pour over the salad just before serving, mix again carefully, and serve immediately.

(I did omit 'Rew' or Rue in the translation to the contemporary version, for it's exceedingly bitter, acrid and nauseous taste could overpower a salad.)

Brotchan Foltchep (Leek and Oatmeal Soup)

This soup probably started out as oatmeal porridge enriched with leeks and milk, and has been eaten in Irish monasteries for over 1400 years.

3 or 4 medium-size leeks, about 1 1/2 pounds

1/4 to 1/2 stick butter (1-2 ounces)

2 cups chicken or vegetable stock

2 cups milk

1/2 cup heavy cream

3/4 cup raw, steel-cut porridge oats

parsley (flat Italian, chopped) for garnishing

salt and white pepper to taste

Wash the leeks well. Trim off the root ends and discard. Starting at the white, root ends, slice the leeks thinly. Place in a deep bowl of cold water, and rub the leeks between your hands, gently, to separate the rings and rinse off any remaining dirt. Remove leek slices and drain and set aside.

In a pot, bring the stock and milk to a simmer. Stir in the oats, bring almost to a boil, and simmer for 20-30 minutes, or until the oats are done.

While the oats are simmering, melt the butter in a saute pan, over low heat. Cook the leeks for five or ten minutes, until they begin to soften, but not brown. When the oats are about half done, add the leeks with their butter to the pot of soup. The leeks and the oatmeal should be done at the same time. Remove from heat, add the cream, and the salt and white pepper to taste. Garnish with the parsley.

Pottage (a Barley and Vegetable Stew)

3 cups water

salt

1 1/2 cup barley, cooked

1 cup finely chopped cabbage

1/2 cup finely chopped onion and/or leek

1 cup chopped spinach

Boil the cabbage, onion/leek and spinach until tender, and drain. Then add the cooked barley, mix and salt to taste.

Vegetable side dishes

The Celtic method of selecting vegetables for the evening meal was solely based on what was available. Throughout the Celtic area as well as including the historic European continent, adding two vegetables together and mashing them was a standard. These combinations include:

Potch Erfyn, a common dish of swedes (turnips) and potatoes;

Stwns pys (potatoes and peas);

Swedes pys (turnips and peas);

Stwns Ffa (potato or turnip and broad beans);

Potatoes and Kale, a traditional Dutch favorite,

and sometimes peas and beans together with melted butter.

Apple Topped Sweet Potatoes

4 medium-size sweet potatoes (about 3 1/2 lbs)

3/4 cup pecans, coarsely chopped

1/4 cup butter

1 large sweet variety apple, coarsely chopped

1/2 cup date sugar

1/2 teaspoon ground cinnamon

1/4 teaspoon ground nutmeg

Wash sweet potatoes, and cut a slit along the top, then place on a baking sheet and bake at 425 degrees F for 1 hour and 15 minutes or until tender. Heat the nuts in a skillet over medium low heat, shaking often, about 5 to 7 minutes or until toasted. Remove the nuts from the hot pan immediately.

Melt the butter in a skillet, add chopped apple and raisins and sauté for 2 to 3 minutes or until the apple is tender. Stir in date sugar, cinnamon, and nutmeg and remove from heat.

Cut sweet potatoes in half and scoop out the pulp with a soup spoon. Place pulp in a baking dish and mash with the back of a fork. Smooth the pulp out into an even layer of uniform thickness. Place apple mixture on top and spread it evenly over the sweet potatoes. Sprinkle with nuts and serve. This recipe is good for saving as well. Simply re-bake until hot, approximately 15 minutes, then serve.

Pea And Roasted Garlic Soup

4 bulbs of garlic (less if you like)

2 onions peeled and roughly chopped

2 T olive oil

1 kg or 2 lbs frozen peas

30 oz good vegetable stock

Sea salt and freshly ground black pepper to taste.

Wrap the garlic in foil and roast at 350 degrees F for 40 minutes or until soft. Fry the onion in oil and a little stock for approx 3 minutes until soft. Add the frozen peas and coat in the oil/stock blend. Add the balance of stock and bring to the boil, reduce the heat and simmer for 5 minutes. Bring the garlic out of the oven and leave to cool for 5 minutes, cut the top off and squeeze the soft roasted garlic into the pea soup, puree roughly.

You can serve with a dollop of sour cream or yogurt and a sprinkling of chives.

Salmon and Pea Crustless Pie

20 oz cooked salmon, skinned

1 cup low fat milk

grated rind of 1 lemon

12 oz frozen peas

2 shallots, peeled and finely chopped

3 T chives, finely chopped

Sea salt and black pepper

Preheat the oven to 200°C/400°F. Peel the potatoes, cut into bite size chunks, add enough water, just to cover the potatoes and put to boil. Lower the heat to simmer and cook the potatoes until tender. Drain the potatoes in a colander, return them to the pan and mash them, adding the milk and season with sea salt and black pepper, set aside.

Remove the salmon, strain and when the fish is cool enough to handle, flake the fish.

Mix the cooked salmon, grated lemon rind, peas, shallots and chives, season with sea salt and black pepper. Place the fish mixture in a greased or sprayed ovenproof dish, spoon the mashed potato on top covering surface. Cook in the oven for 25 minutes and serve.

Pea and Barley Soup

1 T olive oil

1 medium onion, peeled and chopped

2 medium carrots, diced

1 stick celery, cut into ¼ inch chunks

2 oz (dried weight) of barley or rolled oats

1 clove garlic, peeled and finely chopped

1 sprig fresh thyme, pulled from the stalk (1 tsp of dried)

1 sprig fresh oregano (½ tsp dried)

50 oz good vegetable stock

Sea salt and freshly ground black pepper (optional)

1/2 leek, cut in half lengthways and chopped into ¼ inch chunks

2 cups savoy cabbage, shredded or cubed

10 oz frozen peas

2 T chopped parsley

Fry the chopped onion, carrot, and celery with the barley over a medium heat for one minute. Add the garlic cook for a further one minute. Add the sprig of fresh thyme pulled off the stalk, or half a teaspoon of dried, one sprig fresh oregano (half tsp dried) then the stock. Season with the sea salt and black pepper. Bring to the boil and boil for 12 minutes. Add the leek and cabbage and for a further 5 minutes until they are nearly tender. Then add the parsley and the peas and boil for another 5 minutes. Season to taste and garnish with fresh chives. Serve hot.

Green Pea Hummus

17 oz frozen peas

3 cloves garlic, crushed

3 T light tahini paste/sesame seed paste

juice of 1 large lemon (add more if preferred)

1 tsp ground cumin

1 T olive oil

1/4 tsp chili powder

Sea salt and black pepper

Add the peas to a pan of boiling water and simmer for 3 minutes. Drain the peas and put in a food processor along with all the other ingredients; mix well until a paste is formed. Season with sea salt and black pepper according to taste. Serve the green pea hummus in a dipping bowl with toasted pita bread and raw vegetables.

Peas And Brussels Sprouts With Hazelnuts

6 oz prepared/cooked brussel sprouts

12 oz frozen peas

1 oz butter

2 oz hazelnuts, roughly chopped

zest and juice of one orange

1 tsp sugar

Sea salt and black pepper

Cook the brussel sprouts in boiling, salted water for 5 minutes or until nearly tender, add the peas, bring to the boil and simmer for a further 2 minutes. Drain and place into a warm serving dish.

Meanwhile, melt the butter in a small heavy based frying pan. When the butter is melted, add the chopped nuts and fry for one minute until slightly golden. Add the orange juice and the sugar and boil for a further minute. Add the grated orange zest. Season with a little black pepper and pour over the vegetables.

Split Pea Soup

2 cups split peas, rinsed

6 cups cold water

5 cups broth

1 carrot, finely chopped

1 celery stalk with leaves, finely chopped

1 onion, finely chopped

3 garlic cloves, finely chopped

1 teaspoon sugar (optional)

2 teaspoons lemon juice

salt & pepper to taste

dash each of parsley, thyme, marjoram and cayenne pepper

In a large pot add peas with 6 cups of cold water. Bring the water to a boil, then reduce the heat and simmer for 1 1/2 hours until the split peas are tender.

Add chicken broth, carrot, celery, onion, garlic, sugar, lemon juice, and all spices. Bring to a boil, reduce heat and simmer for another 1/2 hour or until carrots are soft. Cool slightly, then puree in a blender for a smooth soup, or eat as is.

Sorrel Soup

Although Sorrel was used culturally, the sorrel is known to aggravate previously undiagnosed conditions related to rheumatic-type complaints, kidney or bladder stones.

A little history about Sorrel soup. It was a simple soup made from water, sorrel leaves and salt. Other possible ingredients are egg yolks or boiled eggs and boiled potatoes. It is known in Russian, Polish, Lithuanian and Eastern European Jewish cuisines. Its other English names are spelled variously; *schav, shchav, shav, shtshav*, are borrowed via Yiddish language derived from the Polish name *szczaw* for sorrel. It is often served cold with sour cream.

It is characterized by its sour taste due to oxalic acid present in sorrel (called "sorrel acid" in Slavic languages). The "sorrel-sour" taste may disappear when sour cream is added, as the oxalic acid would react with calcium and casein.

In Polish, Ukrainian, and Russian cuisines sorrel soup may be prepared using any kind of broth instead of water and may be served either hot or chilled. Otherwise it may be a kosher food.

Nuts, Oils and Vinegars

More beneficial ingredients to add! Sometimes it's not just the food, it's what you add to it. These following items are going to improve your food nutritionally, and help add to the benefits of the Celtic foods that you will be preparing.

Vinegar

Vinegar is a sour-tasting liquid made from the oxidation of ethanol in wine, cider, beer, fermented fruit juice, or nearly any other liquid containing alcohol. Commercially available vinegar usually has a pH of about 2.4. There are many types of vinegars to chose from. I personally have a bottle of pasteurized apple cider vinegar that I love to add to certain foods. From making your own salad dressings to drizzling on broccoli and potatoes, find some great ways to add vinegar to your diet plan to aid in your success.

The word Vinegar comes from the Old French *vin aigre,* meaning "sour wine." It has been used since ancient times, and is an important element in traditional cuisines of the world. So-called "white vinegar", which is transparent, can be made by oxidizing a distilled alcohol. Alternatively, it may be nothing more than a solution of acetic acid in water which can still be used for culinary as well as cleaning purposes.

Malt vinegar is made by malting barley, causing the starch in the grain to turn to maltose. An ale is then brewed from the maltose and allowed to turn into vinegar, which is then aged. A cheaper alternative, called "non-brewed condiment," is a solution of 4-8% acetic acid colored with caramel. There is also around 13% citric acid present. Britons commonly use malt vinegar on chips; it may be used in other territories where British-style fish and chips are served.

Wine vinegar is made from red or white wine, and is the most commonly used vinegar in Mediterranean countries, Germany, and other countries. As with wine, there is a considerable range in quality. Better quality wine vinegars are matured in wood for up to two years and exhibit a complex, mellow flavor. There are more expensive wine vinegars made from individual varieties of wine, such as Champagne vinegar and sherry vinegar.

Fruit vinegars are made from fruit wines without any additional flavoring. Common flavors of fruit vinegar include black currant, raspberry, and quince. Typically, the flavors of the original fruits remain taste-able in the final vinegar.

Most such vinegars are produced in Europe, where there is a growing market for high price vinegars made solely from specific fruits, as opposed to non-fruit vinegars which are infused with fruits or fruit flavors. Persimmon vinegar is a new and becoming popular vinegar.

Balsamic vinegar is an aromatic, aged type of vinegar manufactured in Modena, Italy, from the concentrated juice of Trebbiano white grapes. Its flavor is rich, sweet, and complex, with the finest grades being the end product of years of aging in a successive number of casks made of various types of wood (including oak, mulberry, chestnut, cherry, juniper, ash, and acacia). Originally an artisanal product available only to the Italian upper classes, balsamic vinegar became widely known and available around the world in the late 20th century. This particular vinegar is very popular as a salad and coleslaw dressing and can come in fruit flavors.

Rice Vinegar. The Japanese prefer a more delicate rice vinegar and use it for much the same purposes as Europeans, as well as for sushi rice, in which it is an essential ingredient. Rice vinegar is available in white, red, and black variants. Black rice vinegar may be used as a substitute for balsamic vinegar, though its dark color and the fact that it is aged may be the only similarity between the two products. Some types of rice vinegar are sweetened or otherwise seasoned.

Coconut vinegar, made from the sap of the coconut palm, is used extensively in Southeast Asian cuisine, particularly in the Philippines, as well as in some cuisines of India. A cloudy white liquid, it has a particularly sharp, acidic taste with a slightly yeasty note.

Cane vinegar, made from sugar cane juice, is most popular in the Philippines although it is also produced in France and the United States. It ranges from dark yellow to golden brown in color and has a mellow flavor, similar in some respects to rice vinegar, though with a somewhat "fresher" taste. Although created from the sugar cane, it is not sweeter than other vinegars, containing no residual sugar.

Raisin Vinegar made from raisins is used in cuisines of the Middle East, and is produced in Turkey. It is cloudy and medium brown in color, with a mild flavor.

Honey Vinegar made from honey is rare, though commercially available honey vinegars are produced in Italy and France.

Chinese black vinegar is an aged product made from rice, wheat, millet, or sorghum. It has an inky black color and a complex flavor.

Popular **fruit-flavored vinegars** include those infused with whole raspberries, blueberries, or figs. Some of the more exotic fruit-flavored vinegars include blood orange and pear. Make sure that your fruit flavored vinegar contains actual fruit and not a synthetic fruit flavor, natural is always better.

Herb vinegars are flavored with herbs, most commonly Mediterranean herbs such as thyme or oregano. Such vinegars can be prepared at home by adding sprigs of fresh or dried herbs to store-bought vinegar. An East Asian variety of flavored vinegar known as sweetened vinegar is made from rice wine and herbs including ginger, cloves and other spices. It is an integral ingredient in the traditional Chinese postnatal health and celebratory dishes.

Apple cider vinegar, sometimes known simply as cider vinegar, is made from cider or apple juice, and is often sold unfiltered, with a brownish-yellow color; it often contains mother of vinegar. It is currently very popular, partly due to its alleged beneficial health and beauty properties. Some countries, like Canada, prohibit the selling of vinegar over a certain percentage of acidity.

In terms of cooking, cider vinegar is not usually suitable for use in delicate sauces, but is excellent for use in chutneys and marinades. It is used to make vinegar pie and can also be used to pickle foods, but will darken light fruits and vegetables.

Medicinal benefits. Hippocrates prescribed vinegar for many ailments, from skin rash to ear infection. Vinegar is a folk medicine used in China to prevent the spread of virus such as SARS (Severe Acute Respiratory Syndrome) and other pneumonia outbreaks.

The therapeutic use of vinegar is even recorded in the second verse of the nursery rhyme "Jack and Jill": "Went to bed and bound his head / With vinegar and brown paper." As with some nursery rhymes, there is truth in the story. This one comes from the village of Kilmersdon in Somerset. The vinegar used would likely have been cider vinegar.

Apple cider vinegar is a much more useful astringent than ice and will reduce inflammation, bruising and swelling in approximately a third of the time that ice will take. Application is directly onto the skin with a flannel, and left on for an hour or so. Vinegar along with hydrogen peroxide (H_2O_2) is used in the livestock industry to kill bacteria and viruses before refrigeration storage. A chemical mixture of peracetic acid is formed when acetic acid is mixed with hydrogen peroxide. It is being used in some Asian countries by aerosol sprays for control of pneumonia. A mixture of five-percent acetic acid and three-percent hydrogen peroxide is commonly used.

Apple cider vinegar is often touted as a medical aid, from cancer prevention to alleviation of joint pain to weight loss. These claims began in Biblical times, and more recently in 1958, when Dr. D.C. Jarvis made the remedy popular with a book that sold 500,000 copies.

Claims that cider vinegar can be used as a beauty aid also persist, despite the fact that apple cider vinegar can sometimes be very dangerous to the eyes. The acid will burn and the eyes will become red, but no damage to the eyes has ever been described. If the vinegar contains *mother of vinegar,* the slime bacteria of the mother can cause ophthalmitis. Many believe that vinegar is also a cure to mild to moderate sunburn when soaked on the area with a towel or in a bath.

Cider vinegar is also claimed to be a solution to dandruff, in that the acid in the vinegar kills the fungus Malassezia furfur (formerly known as Pityrosporum ovale) and restores the chemical balance of the skin.

Two tablespoons of vinegar before a meal was found to prevent blood sugar spikes in a study by Arizona State University.

✔uts

Hazelnuts. In 1995, evidence of large-scale Mesolithic nut processing, some 9,000 years old, was found in a midden pit on the island of Colonsay in Scotland. The evidence consists of a large, shallow pit full of the remains of hundreds of thousands of burned hazelnut shells. Hazelnuts have been found on other Mesolithic sites, but rarely in such quantities or concentrated in one pit. The nuts were radiocarbon dated to 7720+/-110BP, which calibrates to circa 7000 BC. Similar sites in Britain are known only at Farnham in Surrey and Cass ny Hawin on the Isle of Man.

This discovery gives an insight into communal activity and planning in the period. The nuts were harvested in a single year and pollen analysis suggests that the hazel trees were all cut down at the same time. The scale of the activity, unparalleled elsewhere in Scotland, and the lack of large game on the island, suggests the possibility that Colonsay contained a community with a largely vegetarian diet for the time they spent on the island. The pit was originally on a beach close to the shore, and was associated with two smaller stone-lined pits, whose function remains obscure, a hearth, and a second cluster of pits.

Hazelnuts have a significant place among the types of dried nut in terms of nutrition and health because of the special composition of fats (primarily oleic acid), protein, carbohydrates, vitamins (vitamin E), minerals, dietary fibers, phytosterol (beta-cytosterol) and antioxidant phenolics. The nutritional and sensory properties of hazelnut make it a unique and ideal material for food products. Hazelnuts are a good source of energy with their 60.5% fat content.

Oils

Flax, Seeds and Oil

The nutritional value of flax includes complex carbohydrates, natural sugars, fibres, fat, protein, thiamine, riboflavin, niacin, pantothenic acid, vitamin B6, Vitamin C, calcium, iron, magnesium, phosphorus, potassium, and zinc.

Flax seeds come in two basic varieties, brown and yellow or golden, and have similar nutritional characteristics and equal amounts of short-chain omega-3 fatty acids. Although brown flax can be consumed as readily as yellow, and has been for thousands of years, it is better known as an ingredient in paints, fibre and cattle feed.

One tablespoon of ground flax seeds and three tablespoons of water may serve as a replacement for one egg in baking by binding the other ingredients together. Ground flax seeds can also be mixed in with oatmeal, yogurt or any other food item where a nutty flavor is appreciated. Flax seed sprouts are edible, with a slightly spicy flavor. Roasted flax seed can be, and has been, powdered and eaten with boiled rice, a little water, and a little salt since ancient times. It is aromatic and considered soothing for the stomach, useful as a laxative, and good for health.

Flax seeds are chemically stable while whole, and milled flax seed can be stored at least 4 months at room temperature with minimal or no changes in taste, smell, or chemical markers of rancidity. But ground flaxseed can go rancid at room temperature in as little as one week. Refrigeration and storage in sealed containers will keep ground flax from becoming rancid for a longer period of time.

The reported health benefits of flax seeds are related to their high levels of lignans and Omega-3 fatty acids. Lignans may benefit the heart, possess anti-cancer properties and studies performed found reduced growth in specific types of tumors. Flax seed may also lower cholesterol levels, and benefit individuals with certain types of cancers. However, the Mayo Clinic reports that the alpha linolenic acid in flaxseed may be associated with higher risk of prostate cancer, and cautions that those with, or at risk for, prostate cancer should not take flaxseed.

Flax may also lessen the severity of diabetes by stabilizing blood-sugar levels. There is some support for the use of flax seed as a laxative due to its dietary fibre content, though excessive consumption without liquid can result in intestinal blockage, because the flax will absorb liquids in the intestinal tract.

Flax is the emblem of Northern Ireland and used by the Northern Ireland Assembly. In a coronet, it appeared on the reverse of the British one pound coin to represent Northern Ireland on coins minted in 1986 and 1991. Flax also represents Northern Ireland on the badge of the Supreme Court of the United Kingdom and on various logos associated with it.

Olive Oil

The greatest example of a monounsaturated fat is olive oil, and it is a major component of the Mediterranean Diet. Olive oil is a natural juice which preserves the taste, aroma, vitamins and properties of the olive fruit. Olive oil is the only vegetable oil that can be consumed as it is—freshly pressed from the fruit.

The beneficial health effects of olive oil are due to both its high content of monounsaturated fatty acids and its high content of antioxidative substances. Studies have shown that olive oil offers protection against heart disease by controlling LDL ("bad") cholesterol levels while raising HDL (the "good" cholesterol) levels. No other naturally produced oil has as large an amount of monounsaturated as olive oil—mainly oleic acid.

Olive oil is very well tolerated by the stomach. In fact, olive oil's protective function has a beneficial effect on ulcers and gastritis. Olive oil activates the secretion of bile and pancreatic hormones much more naturally than prescribed drugs, and consequently, it lowers the incidence of gallstone formation.

Studies have shown that people who consumed about 2 tablespoons of virgin olive oil daily for 1 week showed less oxidation of LDL cholesterol and higher levels of antioxidant compounds in their blood.

Olive oil is clearly one of the good oils, one of the healing fats, containing the critical omega 6 to omega 3 ratio AND omega-9.

Spanish researchers suggest that including olive oil in your diet may prevent colon cancer. Laboratory studies showed that a diet supplemented with olive oil had a lower risk of colon cancer than with a safflower oil-supplemented diets.

Generally, olive oil is extracted by pressing or crushing olives. Olive oil comes in different varieties, depending on the amount of processing involved. Varieties include:

Extra virgin—considered the best, least processed, comprising the oil from the first pressing of the olives.

Virgin—from the second pressing.

Pure—undergoes some processing, such as filtering and refining.

Extra light—undergoes considerable processing and only retains a very mild olive flavour.

When buying olive oil you will want to obtain a high quality Extra Virgin oil. The oil that comes from the first "pressing" of the olive, is extracted without using heat (a cold press) or chemicals, and has no "off" flavors is awarded "extra virgin" status. The less the olive oil is handled, the closer to its natural state, the better the oil. If the olive oil meets all the criteria, it can be designated as "extra virgin".

"Pure" olive oil is made by adding a little extra virgin olive oil to refined olive oil. It is a lesser grade oil that is also labeled as just "olive oil" in the U.S.

"Light" olive oil is a marketing concept and not a classification of olive oil grades. It is completely unregulated by any certification organizations and therefore has no real precedent to what its content should be. Sometimes, the olive oil is cut with other vegetable oils.

Keep olive oil in a cool and dark place, tightly sealed, as heat and light will promote rancidity. Like other oils, olive oil is like other oils and can easily go rancid when exposed to air, light or high temperatures.

There is some research that states that Canola oil is a good substitute for olive oil, due to its concentration of monounsaturated fatty acids. Olive oil is far superior and has been around for thousands of years. Canola oil is a relatively recent development and the original crops were unfit for human consumption due to their high content of a dangerous fatty acid called euric acid. This is the type of oil that virtually all fast food restaurants use.

If the taste of olive oil is a problem, or if you are frying or sautéing food, then you should consider coconut oil. Many nutritionally misinformed people would consider this unwise due to coconut oil's nearly exclusive content of saturated fat. However, this is just not the case. Because it has mostly saturated fat, it is much less dangerous to heat. The heat will not tend to cause the oil to transition into dangerous trans fatty acids.

Coconut Oil

Coconut Oil was not readily available back in the old Celtic days, but we are incorporating the benefits of the past with the proven benefits of today. And Coconut Oil has recently be touted to be one of the best oils that can be used for a wide variety of purposes.

The health benefits of coconut oil include hair care, skin care, stress relief, maintaining cholesterol levels, weight loss, increased immunity, proper digestion and metabolism, relief from kidney problems, heart diseases, high blood pressure, diabetes, HIV and cancer, dental care, and bone strength. These benefits of coconut oil can be attributed to the presence of lauric acid, capric acid and caprylic acid, and its properties such as antimicrobial, antioxidant, antifungal, antibacterial, soothing, etc.

The uniqueness of lauric acid is that the human body converts it into monolaurin which is claimed to help in dealing with viruses and bacteria causing diseases such as herpes, influenza, cytomegalovirus, and even HIV. It helps in fighting harmful bacteria such as listeria monocytogenes and heliobacter pylori, and harmful protozoa such as giardia lamblia.

As great as coconut oil is for your insides, it is just as good on the outsides. Coconut oil is one of the best natural nutrition for hair. It helps in healthy growth of hair providing them a shiny complexion. Regular massage of the head with coconut oil ensures that your scalp is free of dandruff, lice, and lice eggs, even if your scalp is dry. It is an excellent conditioner and helps in the re-growth of damaged hair. It also provides the essential proteins required for nourishing damaged hair. Apply it topically for hair care.

Coconut oil is very soothing and it helps in removing stress. Apply coconut oil to the head followed by a massage.

Tropical countries have been using this emollient oil since prehistory. Coconut oil is excellent massage oil for the skin, a moisturizer on all types of skins, delays wrinkles, treats various skin problems including psoriasis, dermatitis, eczema and other skin infections. When applied on infections, it forms a chemical layer which protects the infected body part from external dust, air, fungi, bacteria and virus. Coconut oil is most effective on bruises as it speeds up the healing process by repairing damaged tissues. Today, in skin products, coconut oil forms the basic ingredient of various body care products such as soaps, lotions, creams.

There is a misconception spread among many people that coconut oil is not good for the heart. This is because it contains a large quantity of saturated fats. However, coconut oil is beneficial for the heart. It contains about 50% lauric acid, which helps in preventing various heart problems including high cholesterol levels and high blood pressure. The saturated fats present in coconut oil are not harmful as it happens in case of other vegetables oils.

Coconut oil will help in a weight loss plan. It is also easy to digest and it helps in healthy functioning of the thyroid and enzymes systems. Further, it increases the body metabolism by removing stress on the pancreas, thereby burning out more energy and helping obese and overweight people reduce their weight. Hence, people living in tropical coastal areas, who eat coconut oil daily as their primary cooking oil, are normally not fat, obese or overweight.

Dairy

The Celtic Diet would be amiss if the descriptions of some of the historic and Celtic famous cheeses were not mentioned. Although you may not be able to find some of these varieties, there are so many great and flavorful cheeses from around the world that need to be tasted. Add some of these or similarly different cheeses to your day to add that variety we all need. Historically, goats and sheep were often the milk source for a lot of the early cheeses, and certainly worth a try today. This Celtic program is also about eating naturally, and the Celts did just that and in moderation, so go ahead and have some of that real cream and butter too.

Again, it may be a good idea to find cheeses and other dairy products that are created from animals that are not subjected to bulking and synthetic hormones that leech into the same dairy products that are mainstream. Canadian cheese doesn't, and never did, have growth hormones fed to their dairy cows. Check labels carefully, read between the lines.

Archaeologists have found solid evidence of cheese making traditions tracing back as far as 6000 BC, when cow and goat's milk cheeses were stored in tall jars. In 5000 BC Switzerland, milk-curdling vessels have been dug up on Lake Neufchatel. In ancient Babylonia, Sumerians from 3500 BC were depicted with the milking and curdling of cow's milk. Egypt's tomb murals from 2000 BC show butter and cheese were made and stored in skin bags suspended from poles.

The Celtic Nations northern geography and temperamental climate once restricted local cheese artisans to a rather short cheese-making season. The cheeses they produced had to withstand long winters and storing periods and hence, most traditional Scottish cheeses are of the hard, matured variety. Since the advances of refrigeration and temperature-controlled facilities, cheese production has expanded across the country and the seasons. From small creameries to commercial manufacturers, Scotland now boasts more than two dozen cheese producers. And though the ever-popular Scottish Cheddar accounts for about 75% of total production, modern cheeses crafted by artisans and family farmhouse makers are also tempting the taste buds of all cheese eaters.

Cheese

Bonchester, a modern farmhouse cheese, is made from the unpasteurized milk of Jersey cows. Slightly chalky when newly made yet takes on a soft, custard-like consistency when aged for a few weeks. This rich cheese is a past medal winner in the British Cheese Awards.

Caboc (Ross-Shire) is a Scottish cream cheese, made with double cream or cream-enriched milk. According to legend, the tradition of coating Caboc in oatmeal started as an accident. A cattle herder stored the day's cheese in a box which he had used to carry his oatcakes earlier that day. Apparently, the oatmeal-coated cheese was enjoyed so much that from that day, Caboc has been made with an oaten coating.

This rennet-free cheese is formed into a log shape and rolled in toasted pinhead oatmeal, to be served with oatcakes or dry toast. The texture is smooth, slightly thicker and grainier than clotted cream while the color is a pale primrose yellow. The fat content is typically 67-69%, which is comparable with rich continental cream cheeses such as mascarpone. Historically, it was a cheese for the wealthy, unlike the similar Crowdie, which is made from the by-products of skimming cream from milk and thus a poor man's cheese.

Caboc is Scotland's oldest cheese, dating from the 15th century in the Scottish Highlands. According to an ancient recipe, this fresh cow's cheese is made with cream-enriched milk and ripened for just five days. The result is a soft double cream log with a fat content of 69%. Rolled in toasted oatmeal, the cheese offers a combination of nutty, yeasty flavor and sharp, lemony tang. A favorite for spreading on crackers or oatcakes, Caboc is also a nice selection and sold under the seal of Highland Fine Cheeses Ltd.

Crowdie (Gruth). The Vikings introduced this soft fresh cheese to Scotland in the eighth century. Made from skimmed cow's milk, it's naturally low in fat with a creamy yet crumbly texture. Crowdie offers a nice lemony tang that's favored for cooking and eating with oatcakes. Sold in logs or tubs, the vegetarian cheese comes in several versions, including plain, peppercorn, garlic and herb.

Dunsyre Blue is a very creamy and sweet, mild blue cheese made from the unpasteurized milk of Ayrshire cows. When aged, chunks of blue-green mould spice the smooth, creamy interior, and a variety of moulds can also be seen on the moist white rind. The cylinder-shaped cheese is usually wrapped in foil and is suitable for vegetarians.

Isle of Mull Cheddar. This hard cow's milk cheese is made on the Isle of Mull off Scotland's west coast. This cylindrical artisan cheese is firm pressed, wrapped in cloth and matured for 12 months in the dairy's cellar. It's uniqueness in character is often compared to a fine malt, with a pale color and tangy, spicy, malted barley flavors. Though the texture is slightly grainy and softer than a traditional English Cheddar, the flavor is quite deep and powerful. At a full and rich maturity, the cheese sometimes develops blue veins—a delicious natural perk. Isle of Mull Cheddar also comes with herbs, caraway seeds and peppers.

Lanark Blue. Sometimes called "Scotland's Roquefort" this famous sheep's milk blue is handmade in a farmhouse creamery. Sprinkled with mould before curdling, the cheese is slightly sweet and streaked with green-blue veins throughout. Lanark Blue is molded into rounds, wrapped in foil and matured for three months.

Orkney Extra Mature Cheddar. Made on the island of Orkney, this traditional creamery cheese is a favorite all over Britain. Hard, nutty and creamy in flavor, and offering a delicious hint of burnt onion. The block-shaped Cheddar is typically aged between 15 and 18 months, displaying tiny crystals of calcium lactate when aged.

Seriously Strong Cheddar. This strong and savory cheese is made with pasteurized cow's milk from the finest farms in Dumfries and Galloway. Hard, yet moist in texture, it has a distinctive, biting flavor that hints of caramel and butterscotch. Seriously Strong Cheddar is suitable for vegetarians and is excellent for eating out of hand, melting, grilling and grating too. A version colored with annatto is famous in Scotland, while the white variety is more popular in England. This cheese is the UK's best-selling Cheddar.

Crowdie is a Scottish cream cheese. It is often eaten with oatcakes, and recommended before a ceilidh (Scottish party) as it is said to alleviate the effects of whisky-drinking. The texture is soft and crumbly, the taste slightly sour. Like cottage cheese it is very low in fat, being made from skimmed milk.

Dunlop cheese is a mild cheese which resembles a soft Cheddar cheese in texture. It is a well-known cheese originating in Scotland. It was first made in south western Scotland in the 18th century.

What about Welsh cheeses? They're so good they were once used as part of divorce settlements. Under the laws of Welsh ruler

Hywel Dda, cheeses that were washed in brine went to the wife, and cheeses that were hung up went to the husband. Wales has a long-standing tradition for producing delicious, high-quality cheeses. The earliest varieties resembled the present day Caerphilly, but they were made from goat and sheep's milks and immersed in brine. Later, in the 17th and 18th centuries, cow's milk became the cheese-making ingredient of choice.

By the early 20th century, the production of Caerphilly moved to England because the demand for the cheese outgrew its Welsh production. Unfortunately, by the time of WWII, cheese making in Wales had come to a near standstill—many of the small Welsh cheese producers were run out of business by the larger English factories.

Some interesting cheese facts:

- Cheddar is named after the Cheddar Gorge caves in Somerset where the cheese used to be stored to ripen. Cheddar is one of the most widely made cheeses in the world.

- Shropshire Blue is not actually made in Shropshire, but Derbyshire, Leicestershire and Nottinghamshire.

- Cheshire is one of the oldest British cheeses, and even gets a mention in the Domesday Book.

- Cornish Yarg came from a recipe found in a book in a farmer's attic—his name was Mr. Gray (Yarg spelt backwards!)

- Caerphilly was traditionally eaten by Welsh coal miners for their lunch.

All the natural goodness that is found in cheese, is also found in other dairy products. The main point when adding dairy to your Celtic health plan is to be sure to avoid dairy that contains growth hormones. It is these growth hormones that are fed to the animals that keep them large and overweight, that you are getting as well.

Butter

One of the things that people don't like about butter is that it is hard. If you want to butter a slice of bread, it may tear it. There is a solution. You can allow the butter to soften at room temperature, add approximately equal amounts of extra virgin olive oil, and gently mix. Then when you get the butter from the fridge, it is spreadable. When shopping, get salted or unsalted, and check the label for colorants, you don't need those either.

Cream

A little cream goes a long way, in your drinks or an a dessert of berries. Select a lower fat version and use sparingly in your meals.

Eggs

Research has shown that eating a well-balanced breakfast can improve concentration level and attention span, math and reading skills, behaviour, and test scores.

Eggs are packed with 14 essential nutrients that you need to stay healthy and active. One large egg contains just 5 grams of fat and only 70 calories.

The protein in eggs can help you lose weight by controlling the rate at which your body absorbs calories. A recent study compared an egg-based breakfast to a bagel-based breakfast, each containing the same number of calories. Those who ate eggs for breakfast ate fewer calories at lunch, felt less hungry and ate up to 400 less calories over a 24-hour period.

Choline, a substance found in egg yolks, stimulates brain development and function. Choline has been recognized as an essential nutrient, but is not produced by our body in adequate amounts. Two large eggs provide an adult with the recommended daily intake of choline.

Eggs help to keep your eyes healthy. Lutein and zeaxanthin are antioxidants found in egg yolks and are believed to help protect eyes against damage due to ultraviolet radiation from the sun.

Including protein-rich eggs in your meals and snacks helps sustain your energy level and curb hunger, cravings and unhealthy snacking.

Protein is the most filling nutrient. It helps control the rate at which calories are absorbed by your body.

Eggs are one of the few foods considered to be a complete protein. A complete protein contains the nine essential amino acids your body cannot produce naturally. The amino acids help form protein and are vital to your body's health.

In addition to supplying energy for your body to function, protein is essential for building and repairing tissue and keeping your body strong and healthy. Muscles, organs, skin and hair, as well as antibodies, enzymes and hormones are all made from protein. Protein also helps fight infections, keeps body fluids in balance and helps your body maintain a healthy metabolism.

Milk

Choose a 2% or 1% or skim in order to avoid too much fat in our diet. Try to limit yourself to no more than 2 cups a day. Consider a Rice, Almond or Soy milk.

Ice Cream?

No more than ¼ cup for now. Ice cream is a lot of cream and a lot of sugar. You can have more later after you have reached your goal.

Yogurt

Yogurt is more than just milk. It has more calcium and protein because of the added cultures, as well as being a great source of protein, calcium, roboflavin and vitamin B 12. One of yogurt's greatest benefits is its active and living cultures. These microorganisms are responsible for many health and nutritional benefits, specifically our intestinal tract, which improves the entire body.

There are three types of yogurt: regular (whole milk), low-fat and skim. Low-fat and skim yogurt are good for people who are on a cholesterol lowering diet or just simply watching their weights. These types of yogurt do not raise blood cholesterol levels.

Some people have trouble digesting lactose, a carbohydrate in milk and milk products, because of the deficiency of enzyme lactase in the body. Live yogurt cultures produce lactase and break down the lactose. Yogurt is a healthy way to get the calcium the body needs, for the people who can not tolerate milk products.

Other benefits of live and active cultures in the yogurt are that they may help to boost the immune system. They encourage the right kind of bacteria to multiply in the gut. These bacteria help to digest food and prevent stomach infections. Also, they help to provide relief from vaginal infections.

Yogurt is a fresh dairy product that must be stored in the refrigerator. The heat treated yogurt has a longer shelf life but it does not give the nutritional benefits like the yogurt with live cultures because heat processing destroys the cultures. To get the most health benefit from yogurt, there must be a live and active cultures seal on the label.

Mediterranean countries use a lot of yogurt in their cuisine. They usually eat yogurt, plain with no sugar, along with main dishes like stuffed cabbage and spinach. They add yogurt to their salads or use it to make traditional *"meze"*. They also prepare yogurt drinks made with plain yogurt, salt and water and serve it with shish kebabs. Fried vegetables such as eggplant or zucchini are eaten with yogurt. Cucumber and yogurt salad is very popular among the Mediterranean countries, it is prepared with yogurt, cucumbers, fresh or dried mint, garlic and salt.

To add more yogurt to everyday diet, here are some healthier alternatives and tips:

-Replace mayonnaise and salad dressings with yogurt;

-Replace ice cream and milkshakes with frozen yogurt and mixed fruit yogurt smoothies;

-Make dips with yogurt instead of sour-cream;

-Try using yogurt cheese instead of cream cheese.

Cottage Cheese

Cottage cheese is one of the most versatile cheeses around, and with its soft texture and rather mild taste it's an easy food for almost anyone to enjoy. This soft cheese earns its name from the fact that it was originally made in small cottages as a way to use leftover milk. In addition to being versatile, cottage cheese can be a nutritious addition to almost any diet.

Even four percent milk fat cottage cheese is low in calories with about 120 calories per serving, but you can also buy low fat and fat-free versions which only have around eighty calories. Standard cottage cheese has anywhere from four to six grams of fat, while the fat-free is completely free of fat, although fat-free may have added starches to compensate. Because cottage cheese is filling, a single serving of this low calorie food can be quite satisfying.

The protein of a single serving of cottage cheese has up to fifteen grams of protein, much of it in the form of casein, a slow digesting form of protein. Although not as high in protein as meat and poultry, it's one of the best non-meat sources of protein around. The high protein content of cottage cheese and its high casein content make it a high satiety food so it reduces hunger for longer periods of time.

And better yet, most cottage cheese is low in carbohydrates with carb contents ranging from three grams to six grams. The low fat versions are often higher in carbs since they have added starches.

And it is a good source of calcium, important not only for building strong bones, but also for maintaining normal blood pressure. With around seventy grams per serving, cottage cheese can go a long ways towards meeting the daily calcium quota.

With its versatility, cottage cheese can be used as a healthy, low fat substitute for other higher fat soft cheeses. When pureed in a blender, it can be a base for a healthy and tasty dip. Or have it plain with some herbs and spices to added. Perfect with fruit and as a salad. Use it instead of sour cream on baked potatoes or as a substitute for ricotta cheese in lasagna. Mix it with yogurt or add it into a smoothie.

Soy alternatives

There are soy bean alternatives to every dairy item listed above. If you are avoiding dairy and milk products for any reason, take a good look at your grocers refrigerated sections for soy based items. Or ask at your local health food store.

Dairy Recipes

Some dairy recipes can also be found in the Dessert and Fruit Recipes chapters. Dairy can be quite fattening, so consider using low fat dairy when creating your recipes and preparing your meals. Those extra calories from fat can add up to a couple of pounds worth per week.

Previously mentioned, there is a wide variety of dairy products that you can eat on your plan. From Cottage Cheese and Yogurt, to Eggs and Milk. Select the ones that you will look forward to eating, especially when combined with other Celtic diet foods. And stick to 1/4 to 1/2 cup servings to better ensure success.

Cottage pudding

3 eggs

3/4 cup cream

1 cup small curd cottage cheese

1/2 teaspoon stevia powder

1 teaspoon vanilla extract

Raisins

Nutmeg

Preheat oven to 325 degrees F. and mix eggs, cream, cottage cheese, and stevia powder with a whisk until blended.

Pour into 4 small serving bowls. Sprinkle a few raisins and sprinkle nutmeg on top. Place the bowls in shallow pan with about 1/2" water in the pan. Bake 30-40 minutes, until a knife comes out clean. Top with stevia sweetened whipped cream.

Here's **a Tart in ymbre** day (Onion and Cheese Pie) recipe from 14th century England.

"Tart in ymbre day. Take and perboile oynouns & erbis & presse out þe water & hewe hem smale. Take grene chese and bray it in a morter, and temper it vp with ayren. Do þerto butter, saffroun & salt, & raisons corauns, & a litel sugur with powdour douce, & bake it in a trap, & serue it forth."

Translation: **Amber Day Tart.** Take and parboil onions and herbs & press out the water & cut them small. Take green (aged) cheese & grind it in a mortar, and mix with eggs. Add butter, saffron, salt, currants, and spices, & bake it in a pie shell, and serve it.

3-4 small onions, chopped

2 bunches of parsley, chopped

1 cup shredded Cheddar cheese (OR 1/2 cup unseasoned bread crumbs)

8 eggs, beaten

1 T melted butter

1/8 tsp saffron

1/2 tsp salt

1/4 cup currants

1/8 tsp each cloves and nutmeg

1 nine-inch pie shell

Optional spices could be 1/2 tsp each of sage, basil, or thyme.

Bake at 350° F for 35-40 minutes or until pastry is brown and filling is set.

Scottish Cheddar Soup

2 onions, thinly sliced

1.5 oz butter

1/3 cup flour

2 1/2 cup stock

2 1/2 cup milk

1 pinch pepper

6 oz scottish cheddar cheese, grated

Melt the butter in a saucepan and cook the onions for a few minutes.
Add the flour and cook for another minute. Stir in the milk and stock,
bring to the boil, season and simmer gently for about 5 minutes.
Add the grated cheese to the soup and simmer until melted.

fruit

Let's start with a recipe taken right from the history books. This is a recipe for Apple Snow, often used as a edible center piece for a banquet (dated 1572 from a Scottish Elizabethan).

> *Dyschefull of Snowe. "Take a pottell of swete thycke creame and the whytes of eyghte egges, and beate them altogether wyth a spone. Then putte them in youre reame and a saucerful of Rosewater, and a dyshe full of Sugar wyth all. Then take a stycke and make it cleane, and then cutte it in the ende foure square, and therwith beate all the aforesayde thynges together, and ever as it ryseth take it of and put it into a Collaunder. This done, take one apple and set it in the myddes of it, and a thicke bushe of Rosemary, and set it in the myddes of the Platter. Then cast your Snowe uppon the Rosemary and fyll your platter therwith. And yf you have wafers caste some in wyth all and thus serve them forthe."*

We know the Celts ate strawberries and raspberries. Blackberries also existed, but it is uncertain if they ate them or not as several of the excavations have not included blackberry seeds. Hazelnuts were also used by the Celts, and because of the large quantities of shell fragments recovered from historic sites, hazelnuts are likely to have been locally available.

Evidence for other tree species such as Bird Cherry, Rowan tree, bramble, and rose are likely to have been used as flavourings and sweeteners, made into drinks or condiments, and eaten fresh.

Fruits were mostly eaten as a dessert, and due to the lack of processed foods and candy bars, the sweetness of these fruits would have been very much dessert-like compared to today's standards.

Feel free to consume in abundance any of the fruits listed below. There are also a few Celtic recipes involving these fruits that also includes whipping cream and sugar. So as wonderful and natural as they sound, this doesn't mean that you can focus your entire new eating plan to these particular dishes. But this does mean that you can have your dessert too!

Berries

Blackberries, strawberries, raspberries. All loaded with natural health giving benefits such as providing polyphenols such as flavonoids, anthocyanins, and tannins found mainly in berry skins and seeds. Berry pigments are high in antioxidants and have the oxygen radical absorbance capacity, or ORAC, that is high among plant foods. Together with good nutrient content, ORAC distinguishes berries into a new category of beneficial foods called **superfruits**.

Apples and Crab-apples

The proverb "An apple a day keeps the doctor away," is a Welsh proverb that dates from the 1800's. Research suggests that apples may reduce the risk of colon cancer, prostate cancer and lung cancer. Compared to many other fruits and vegetables, apples contain relatively low amounts of Vitamin C, but are rich source of other antioxidant compounds. The fibre content, while less than in most other fruits, helps regulate bowel movements and may thus reduce the risk of colon cancer. They may also help with heart disease, weight loss, and controlling cholesterol.

Crabapples carry the same healthy benefits, although are found to be too tart or sour for some. Often these apples are used for making jams and jellies. But don't let that stop you from experimenting with crabapples, they can be made with no sugar using Stevia (read about this in the Contemporary Additions chapter).

Figs

Thought to be native to the Middle East, and one of the first fruits ever to be cultivated. Today, California, Turkey and Greece are the main growers of figs.

Figs tend to be more popular in their dried form because fresh figs are very delicate and tend to deteriorate quickly. When selecting fresh figs, choose those which are plump and tender, have a rich, deep colour, are free from bruises and are not mushy. Ripe figs should not be washed until ready to eat and should be kept covered and refrigerated, where they will remain fresh for approximately two days.

Unripe figs should be kept at room temperature and out of direct sunlight.

Figs are high in natural and simple sugars, minerals and fiber. They contain good levels of potassium, calcium, magnesium, iron, copper and manganese. Dried figs contain an impressive 250mg of calcium per 100g, compared to whole milk with only 118mg.

The health benefits of figs include promoting healthy bowel function due to the high levels of fiber. Figs are amongst the most highly alkaline foods, making them useful in balancing the pH of the body.

Suggestions for adding figs to your diet:

1. Just try one. I was amazed that this little dried fruit could be so soft and sweet inside. I felt like I had just discovered some amazing new candy-like food.

2. Chop and add to your oatmeal

3. Simmer with other fruits in a fruit juice and sprinkle with cinnamon before eating.

4. Make a fig-butter. Boil figs with fruit juice till fully rehydrated then blend till smooth and spread on whole grain breads, crackers, or apple slices.

5. Stuff with feta cheese and chopped almonds.

Sour cherry

Or Prunus cerasus, is a native to Europe and southwest Asia. It is closely related to the wild cherry, but has a fruit that is more acidic and used primarily for cooking. This tree is smaller than the wild cherry, has twiggy branches, and crimson-to-near-black cherries. There are two varieties of the sour cherry: the dark-red morello cherry and the lighter-red amarelle cherry.

Cultivated sour cherries were selected from wild specimens from around the Caspian and Black Seas, and were known to the Greeks in 300 BC. They were also extremely popular with Persians and the Romans who introduced them into Britain long before the 1st century AD.

In Britain, their growing as a farm crop became popular in the 16th century. They became a popular crop amongst Kentish (Scottish) growers, and by 1640 over two dozen named farms were recorded. In the Americas, Massachusetts colonists planted the first sour cherry, 'Kentish Red', when they arrived. Sour cherries, unlike their sweet counterpart, are too sour for some people's tastes to be eaten fresh, although the Europeans regularly ate them fresh. Fresh cherries were commonly used in pies and sauces, and the dried versions used in baking.

There is an old dish entitled **Sour Cherry Soup, or hideg meggyleves**, yet if you read the ingredients, it's really just a light sauce. But we won't let that stop us.

Plums and prunes

A plum is a stone fruit tree and is a member of the rose family. Mature plum fruits may have a dusty-white coating that that gives them an opaque appearance and is easily rubbed off. This is an epicuticular wax coating and is known as "wax bloom".

Plum fruit tastes sweet and/or tart; the skin may be particularly tart. It is juicy and can be eaten fresh or used in jam-making or other recipes. Plum juice can be fermented into plum wine; when distilled, this produces a brandy. Dried plums are generally known as prunes, but more accurately, prunes are a distinct type of plum, and may have predated the plums we know of today. Prunes are also sweet and juicy and contain several antioxidants. Plums and prunes are known for their laxative effect and this been attributed to various compounds present in the fruits, such as dietary fiber, sorbitol, and isatin. Dried prune marketers in the United States have, in recent years, begun marketing their product as "dried plums", due to negative connotations connected with elderly people suffering from constipation.

Prunes are used in cooking both sweet and savory dishes. Stewed prunes can be a dessert or added to a vegetable dish such as *Tzimmes*, a traditional Jewish dish with diced or sliced carrots.

Rose hips

The rose hip, or rose haw, is the pomaceous fruit of the rose plant, that typically is red-to-orange, but might be dark purple to-black in some species. Rose hips begin to form in spring, and ripen in late summer through autumn and have been used as a source of Vitamin C. Rose hips are commonly used as a herbal tea, jam, jelly, syrup, beverage, pie, marmalade and wine. Probably the easiest way to incorporate rose hips into your diet plan is with a herbal tea.

The health benefits of this little fruit are becoming well known, they are:

-high in Vitamin C, with about 1700-2000 mg per 100 g in the dried product, one of the richest plant sources;

-Rose hips contain vitamins C, D and E, essential fatty acids and antioxidant flavonoids;

-Rose hip powder is touted as a remedy for osteoarthritis and rheumatoid arthritis.

-Rose hips are used for colds and influenza.

Rose Hip oil, or Rosa Mosquita Oil, is great as a facial moisturizer, instead of store bought chemical laden moisturizers. With a dampened face cloth, apply a few drops of Rose Hip to all areas of your face for an all natural, quick absorbing, moisturizer.

Bilberries

These berries are found in very acidic, nutrient-poor soils throughout the world. They are closely related to North American wild and cultivated blueberries and huckleberries. One characteristic of bilberries is that they produce single or paired berries on the bush instead of clusters, as the blueberry does.

The fruit is smaller than that of the blueberry and similar in taste. Bilberries are darker in colour, and usually appear near black with a slight shade of blue. While the blueberry's fruit pulp is light green, the bilberry's is red or purple, heavily staining the fingers and lips of consumers eating the raw fruit. The red juice is used by European dentists to show children how to brush their teeth correctly, as any improperly brushed areas will be heavily stained.

Bilberries are extremely difficult to grow and are thus seldom cultivated. Fruits are mostly collected from wild plants growing on publicly accessible lands, notably Finland, Sweden, Norway, Scotland, Wales, Ireland, parts of England. Bilberries can be picked by a berry-picking rake like lingon berries, but are more susceptible to damage due to their being softer and juicier than blueberries, also making them difficult to transport. Because of these factors, the bilberry is only available fresh in gourmet stores, where they can cost up to $37 dollars per lb. Frozen bilberries however are available all year round in most of Europe.

In Ireland, the fruit is known as *fraughan*, from the Irish *fraochán*, and is traditionally gathered on the last Sunday in July, known as Fraughan Sunday.

The fruits can be eaten fresh or made into jams, juices or pies. In France and in Italy, they are used as a base for liqueurs and are a popular flavoring for sorbets and other desserts. In Brittany, they are often used as a flavoring for crêpes.

Its health benefits are reputed to be associated with improvement of night vision. Although the effect of bilberry on night vision is controversial, laboratory studies have provided some evidence that bilberry consumption may inhibit or reverse eye disorders such as macular degeneration. A randomized, double-blind, placebo-controlled clinical trial on 50 patients suffering from senile cataracts showed that a combination of bilberry extract and vitamin E administered for 4 months was able to stop lens opacity progress in 97% of the cataracts.

As a deep blue fruit, bilberries contain high levels of anthocyanin pigments, which have been linked experimentally to lowered risk for several diseases, such as those of the heart and cardiovascular system, eyes and cancer.

In folk medicine, bilberry leaves were used to treat gastro- intestinal ailments, applied topically, or made into infusions. Bilberries are also used as a tonic to prevent some infections and skin diseases.

Grapes

A grape is, botanically, a true berry, and can be eaten raw or used for making jam, juice, jelly, vinegar, drugs, wine, grape seed extracts, raisins, and grape seed oil.

Researchers have discovered that although the French tend to eat higher levels of animal fat, surprisingly the incidence of heart disease remains low in France, a phenomenon named the French Paradox and thought to occur from protective benefits of regularly consuming red wine. Apart from any potential benefits of alcohol itself, including reduced platelet aggregation, vasodilation and resveratrol polyphenols, the grape skin may provide other health benefits. Such as reducing vascular damage, lowering blood pressure, and a beneficial increase in the vasodilator hormone. Grape phytochemicals such as the antioxidant resveratrol, have been positively linked to inhibiting any cancer, heart disease, degenerative nerve disease, viral infections and mechanisms of

Alzheimer's disease. Resveratrol is found in large amounts among grape varieties, primarily in their skins and seeds and have about one hundred times higher concentration than pulp. Fresh grape skin contains about 50 to 100 micrograms of resveratrol per gram.

Grape seed oil from crushed seeds is used in cosmeceuticals and skincare products for many perceived health benefits. Grape seed oil is notable for its high contents of tocopherols (vitamin E), phytosterols, and polyunsaturated fatty acids such as linoleic acid, oleic acid and alpha-linolenic acid. Grape seed oil is another oil being used in lotions, creams and massage oils.

Fruit Recipes

Stuffed figs. Simple yet wonderful. Cut a small incision in the bottom of the fig and stuff with cheese, sometimes soft cheese if preferred. Heat these in the oven or grill to make the cheese warm and soft. You can also adds nuts, either with or without the cheese.

Suggested cheeses are blue cheese, fontina, goat cheese, mozzarella, stilton, and teleme, it's the milder cheese that compliments the sweetness of the figs.

Chocolate covered cherries

1 lb, or less, of cherries

2 oz of natural chocolate, dark

Cooking spray on a cookie sheet, wash the cherries, and place them on a towel to dry. Melt the chocolate slowly in a double boiler, stirring constantly with a wooden spoon, until they are just melted and remove from heat. Holding each cherry by the stem, dip them into the chocolate and place the dipped cherry on the tray. Once done, put the tray in the refrigerator for about 15 minutes so the chocolate will cool and harden. Eat within a couple of hours.

Blueberry Sauce

1/2 tsp stevia concentrate powder

1/8 tsp salt

1 1/2 T cornstarch

1/2 cup water

2 cups blueberries

1 T lemon juice

1/2 T butter

Mix stevia, salt and cornstarch in a saucepan. Place on medium heat and add water, stir until thickens. Add blueberries, lemon juice and butter. Continue to stir as it thickens. Remove from heat, cool, serve over yogurt or cottage cheese or oatmeal.

Sour Cherry Soup

4 cups water

1 tsp liquid stevia OR 1.5 T stevia powder

1 Cinnamon stick

4 cups of sour cherries, pitted

pinch of salt

2 T of water

1 T of Cornstarch or arrowroot powder

¼ cup of cream.

In a large saucepan, bring the 4 cups of water, sugar and cinnamon stick to a boil. Reduce heat to medium-low and simmer, stirring to dissolve the stevia, for about 2-3 minutes. Then add the cherries and a pinch of salt and simmer for another 30-40 minutes. Remove the cinnamon stick.

Stir the cornstarch into the 2 tablespoons of water and then quickly whisk the slurry into the simmering cherries. Simmer for another 2-3 minutes to thicken the soup a little. Pour the soup into a bowl, place into the refrigerator until well chilled. Just before serving, stir in the cream.

Fig Tarts

¼ cup of walnuts

1 cup of figs

1 small package of raisins, optional

5-6 ounces of apple juice

1 T of orange zest

1 T of honey

½ tsp of cinnamon.

Process in a food processor until the mixture is a sticky paste.

Press into a pastry pan and bake at 300 degrees for 30-35 minutes.

Apple Cream

1 1/2 lb apples, peeled, cored & sliced

1 T water

Icing sugar, to taste

3 egg whites

¾ tsp liquid stevia OR 1 T + 1 tsp powder

1 cup whipping cream

Cook the sliced apples with the water until soft, and then rub them through a fine sieve to make a smooth puree. Taste and sweeten with a little stevia if necessary. Leave to get cold, then measure out about 8 oz. In a large clean bowl, beat the egg whites until they stand in soft peaks. Gradually beat in the stevia and continue to beat to a stiff, glossy meringue. Gently fold in the measured apple puree, and then spoon into individual glasses or sundae dishes. Top with swirls of whipped cream.

Mixed Berries

1 cup raspberries

1 cup strawberries

½ cup blackberries

¼ cup chopped hazelnuts

Mix berries together. Sprinkle nuts on top. So simple yet so flavourful and good for you.

Cranachan is a traditional Scottish dessert. Nowadays it is usually made from a mixture of whipped cream, honey, and fresh raspberries topped with toasted oatmeal. Earlier recipes for cranachan or cream-crowdie are more plain, sometimes including whisky and treating the fruit as an optional extra. Modern recipes have a high double cream content, which can be replaced wholly or in part by low fat cream.

A traditional way to serve cranachan is to bring dishes of each ingredient to the table, so that each person can assemble their dessert to taste.

Raspberry Brose

2 oz rolled oats

5 oz double cream

7 oz natural fromage frais, (cream or yogurt)

1 T light soft brown sugar

13 oz fresh raspberries (or thawed frozen)

(1 T Scotch was in the original recipe but contemporarily omitted)

Spread out the oats on a baking sheet and toast them under the grill until lightly browned. Allow them to cool. Then whip the cream in a chilled bowl and when the cream is stiffening, add the cream or yogurt, sugar and most of the toasted oats.

Spoon the raspberries into serving dishes and top with the cream mixture. Sprinkle the reserved oats on top.

Meat, Poultry and Fish

There may be a couple of meat items here that don't seem all that edible. You do not have to eat anything here that you don't want to. Take a look at what the Celts ate and incorporate or modify that to your own tastes. For example, if you only like Cod, then substitute all fish recipes with Cod. For vegetarians, use your preferred type of soy product.

Fish

We know about the fish that were eaten during this period from bones which have been found during archaeological excavations. Some bones have been found while the digging was being carried out, but most bones required the soil samples to be washed through fine meshed sieves back in the laboratory. Some bones come from toilet pits and appear to have been chewed up before being swallowed. It has been possible to discover what kinds of fish were eaten by comparing the bones with those of fish today.

Evidence shows a variety of fish were eaten—herring, salmon and eel as well as some which are not eaten much today such as pike, perch and roach. They seem to have also eaten flounder, whiting, plaice, cod and brown trout too. Shellfish, especially oysters, mussels and cockles, seem to have formed part of many peoples diets. Fish was eaten fresh, but was also preserved for less plentiful times of year. This was done by salting, pickling, smoking and drying.

Eel

Freshwater eels and marine or salt water eels are more commonly today to be used in Japanese cuisine but Eels are also very popular in Chinese cuisine, and are prepared in many different ways. Eel is also popular in Korean cuisine and is seen as a source of stamina for men. The European eel and other freshwater eels are eaten in Europe, the United States, and other places. A traditional English food is jellied eels, although the demand has declined since World

War II. In New Zealand, the longfin eel is a traditional Māori food in New Zealand.

The celts and fishermen everywhere have consumed elvers (eels) as a cheap dish, but environmental changes have reduced eel populations. They are now considered a delicacy and are priced at up to $1,400 per kg in the United Kingdom.

But don't eat one raw, eel blood is toxic to humans and other mammals, but both cooking and the digestive process destroys the toxic protein, which causes a condition similar to anaphylaxis shock. So although the Celts, and almost every other coastal country, has historically consumed eels, I think I will pass.

Salmon

Salmon is a popular food and considered to be healthy due to the fish's high protein, high Omega-3 fatty acids, and high vitamin D content. Salmon is also a source of cholesterol. Farmed salmon may contain high levels of dioxins, PCB (polychlorinated biphenyl) levels may be up to eight times higher in farmed salmon than in wild salmon. Omega-3 content may also be lower, and at different proportions than in wild caught specimens. Omega-3 comes in three types, ALA, DHA and EPA; wild salmon has traditionally been an important source of DHA and EPA, which are important for brain function and structure.

A simple rule of thumb is that the vast majority of Atlantic salmon available on the world market are farmed (greater than 99%), whereas the majority of Pacific salmon are wild-caught (greater than 80%). Farmed Atlantic salmon outnumber wild Atlantic salmon 85-to-1.

Salmon flesh is generally orange to red, although there are some examples of white fleshed wild salmon. The natural colour of salmon results from carotenoid pigments, largely from eating krill and other tiny shellfish. Because consumers have shown a reluctance to purchase white-fleshed salmon, colorants are added to the feed of farmed salmon, because prepared diets do not naturally contain these pigments. These colorants can be chemical or from shrimps, or in the use of dried red yeast, both placed in the feed. Like usual, synthetic colorants are usually used as they are the least expensive. In the farmed vs. wild salmon debate, it appears that it isn't so much the possible PCB contamination, nor the possible lack and balance of omega oils, but that the colorants used to pink-up the salmon are far worse.

Canned salmon in the U.S. is usually wild Pacific catch, though some farmed salmon is available in canned form. Smoked salmon is another popular preparation method, and can either be hot or cold smoked. Lox can refer either to cold smoked salmon or to salmon cured in a brine solution. Traditional canned salmon includes some skin (which is harmless) and bone (which adds calcium). Skinless and boneless canned salmon is also available.

Raw salmon flesh may contain Anisakis nematodes, marine parasites that cause Anisakiasis. Before the availability of refrigeration, the Japanese did not consume raw salmon. Salmon and salmon roe have only recently come into use in making sashimi (raw fish) and sushi.

Herring

Also known as Rollmops. Again, Herring are an important economic fish, and utilized by all coastal countries historically.

Herring has been a staple food source since 3000 B.C. There are numerous ways the fish is served and many regional recipes: eaten raw, fermented, pickled, or cured by other techniques. Herring are very high in the long-chain Omega-3 fatty acids EPA and DHA and a source of vitamin D.

Large Baltic herring slightly exceeds recommended limits with respect to PCB and dioxin. Yet, the health benefits from the fatty acids are possibly more important than the risk from dioxins. Which is debatable, and has not been proven. Some sources point out that cancer-reducing effect of omega-3 fatty acids is statistically stronger than the cancer-causing effect of PCBs and dioxins, but there is lack of scientific evidence to prove this. The contaminant levels also depend on the age of the fish which can be inferred from their size. The not monitored rules seem to state that Baltic herrings larger than 17 cm may be eaten twice a month, while herrings smaller than 17 cm can be eaten freely.

Pickled herring is a delicacy in Europe, and has become a part of Baltic, Scandinavian, German, Eastern Slavic and Jewish cuisine. The methods of pickling being that the herring is cured with salt to extract water, then removing the salt and adding flavorings, typically a vinegar, salt, sugar solution to which ingredients like peppercorn, bay leaves and raw onions are added.

In Scandinavia, once the pickling process is finished it is eaten with dark rye bread, crisp bread, sour cream, or potatoes. This dish is common at Christmas, Easter and Midsummer, where it is eaten with akvavit.

In the Middle Ages the Dutch developed a special treat known in English as soused herring or rollmops.

In Scotland the herring is traditionally filleted and after being coated in seasoned pin-head oatmeal is fried in a pan with butter or oil. This dish is usually served with "crushed" buttered boiled potatoes. A kipper is a split and smoked herring, a bloater is a whole smoked herring and a buckling is a hot smoked herring with the guts removed. All are staples of British cuisine. According to George Orwell in The Road to Wigan Pier, the Emperor Charles V erected a statue to the inventor of bloaters.

Today, in Minnesota, kippered herring is a popular pizza topping.

Meat

Most meat eaten by the Saxons came from animals which had more than one use. Sheep were kept for their wool and meat, cows for their milk, sinews and hides. The horn was used for fastenings, drinking vessels and had many other uses. The hide of a bull was as valuable for its leather as the meat. Even the bone was used for belt ends, needles, knife handles, pins for hair and clothing and even for ice skates! Goats were kept for their milk and meat. Only pigs seem to have been raised purely for their meat. It is not clear whether horses were killed for meat or kept purely as riding animals and beasts of burden. The act of eating horse meat became very much frowned upon, and was regarded as a pagan thing to do, so much so that laws were passed to prevent the habit. Although during times of famine, as occurs today, almost anything is game.

Pigs were important for food because they produce large litters, which would quickly mature and be ready as a food source.

Cows produce ten times more meat than sheep or goats and beef production grew increasingly important as pig numbers decreased. Most adult cattle were female, suggesting dairying was also important.

Sheep and goats always accounted for about 50% of the livestock and are ideal animals, as they can be grazed on land that is unsuitable for cattle and pigs, and they are a multi-purpose animal. A high proportion were killed when young and a large number of these were female. Most adult sheep were altered rams raised mainly for wool. The goats were assumed to be similar to feral goats.

Hens, of course, provided eggs as well as meat for the pot, as did ducks and geese. Their hollow bones were used for musical pipes. Various wild birds were eaten too, such as ducks, plover, grouse, herons and geese. Hares were also caught (there were no rabbits until after the Norman Conquest). Deer were hunted for meat, skins and antler. Wild boar would also be hunted for their meat, with their tusks being an important prize for the hunter. Plenty of roast and boiled meats would have been eaten, lots of milk and cheeses and watercress.

Haggis

Fresh meat was generally considered a luxury except for the most affluent until the late 19th century and chickens were not raised on a large scale until the emergence of town grocers in the 1880s. This now allowed people to exchange surplus goods, like eggs, and for the first time purchase a variety food items to diversify their diet.

Haggis is a dish containing a cow or sheep's 'pluck' (heart, liver and lungs), minced with onion, oatmeal, suet, spices, and salt, mixed with stock, and traditionally simmered in the animal's stomach for approximately three hours. Haggis is also a kind of sausage, or savoury pudding cooked in a casing of sheep's intestine, as sausages are.

Most modern commercial haggis is prepared in a casing rather than an actual stomach. There are also meat-free recipes for vegetarians. True historical Haggis is actually not allowed for sale in the United States, the reason being that traditional Haggis would also contain the lungs of the animals and these are considered to contain too many contaminants to be considered a safe food source. If you are willing, I'm sure the modern day Haggis is just as good.

The haggis is a traditional Scottish dish memorialized as the national dish of Scotland by Robert Burns' poem Address to a Haggis in 1787. Haggis is traditionally served with "neeps and tatties" (turnip and potatoes, boiled and mashed separately) and a "dram" (glass of Scotch whisky).

Meat, Poultry, Fish Recipes

Cawdel of Muskels, Scotland 1390 AD

"Take and seeth muskels; pyke hem clene, and waisshe hem clene in wyne. Take almaundes and bray hem. Take somme of the muskels and grynde hem, and some hewe smale; drawe the muskels yground with the self broth. Wryng the almondes with faire water. Do alle thise togider; do therto verious verjuice and vynger. Take whyte of lekes and perboile hem wel; sryng oute the water and hewe hem smale. Cast oile therto, with oynouns perboiled and mynced smale; do therto powdour fort, safroun and salt a lytel. Seeth it, not to stondying, and messe it forth."

A successful diet is one that is simple to buy for and to make. Remember to make any meat servings no larger than the palm of your hand, this will give you approximately 4 oz of protein.

Muscle and Leek Broth (a contemporary version)

Consider using any type of fish for this recipe.

3 lb fresh mussels

1 small onion, finely chopped

4 leeks, thinly sliced

2 T olive oil

1 1/2 oz almonds, ground, optional

2 tsp ginger, ground

pinch Saffron

12 oz fish stock or broth

Salt and pepper to taste

1 T White wine vinegar, or similar

4 T cream.

Prepare muscles with a thorough wash and scrub, remove the beards and discard any mussels that do not close when given a good tap. Place in a large pan and cover with a lid and cook over a high heat for 4 to 5 minutes, shaking the pan until the mussels have opened. Heat the oil in a saucepan and soften the leeks and onions in it for about 3 minutes. Stir in the ground almonds and spices and add the fish stock, stirring well. Let simmer for 25 minutes.

Liquidize the soup and strain through a sieve into a clean saucepan. Taste and season as necessary, and sharpen with wine vinegar. Discard one half of each mussel shell. Reheat the soup and stir in the cream and mussels. Serve hot.

Another type of soup called **Cullen Skink** is a Scottish recipe made of smoked haddock, potatoes and onions and often served as a starter at formal Scottish dinners.

2 small or 1 large Finnan Haddocks filleted

1 large onion, finely chopped

60 oz water

24 oz milk

cooked mashed potato to thicken

2 oz butter

salt and pepper

Garnish: some cream and chopped parsley

Place the fish and onion in water and bring to the boil and simmer gently until the fish is cooked. Remove and flake into pieces. Add potatoes to give a creamy consistency and return the fish to the soup. Garnish with cream and parsley.

Welsh Chicken and Leek Pie

4 lb stewing hen

1 large onion, peeled and quartered

1 small celery stalk, including leaves

a bunch of parsley tied together with one bay leaf

1/4 tsp thyme

1 T salt

10 medium leeks, cut lengthwise then sliced in 1" pieces

1 T finely chopped parsley

rough puff pastry (recipe below)

1 egg yolk combined with 1 T heavy cream

1/4 cup cream

In a 6 to 8 qt pot, combine the chicken, onion, celery stalk, parsley and bay leaf, thyme and salt. Add enough water to cover and bring to the boil. Reduce heat to low and simmer partially covered until tender, about 1 hour. Transfer chicken to a plate, strain the chicken stock, and discarding the herbs. Pour 2 cups of the stock into a saucepan and skim the fat off the surface. Add leeks and bring to the boil. Simmer on low 15 minutes, until leeks are tender.

Cut the meat into 1" pieces, and place evenly in a 1 1/2 qt casserole or baking dish. Pour the leeks and stock over the chicken. Sprinkle with the parsley.

Preheat the oven to 400 degrees F. Roll out the pastry on a lightly floured surface into a rough rectangle 1/4" thick. Then cut two strips, about 12" long and 1/2" wide from the ends. Place the strips around the inside edge of the pan, pressing firmly into place. Moisten them with cold water. Place the remaining pastry over the dish. Trim the excess and crimp the edges together. Cut the remaining pastry into leaf and flower shapes and attach to the top of the pastry with the egg-and-cream mixture. Brush the entire surface also. Cut a 1" round hole in the center, bake for 1 hour, until golden brown. Just before serving, heat the cup of cream to lukewarm and pour it through the hole in the crust.

Rough Puff Pastry

8 oz flour

4 oz butter

1/2 tsp salt

Few drops of lemon juice

Cold water

Sieve the flour and salt into a bowl; add the lemon juice and the butter broken into pieces the size of a walnut; add sufficient cold water to bind the ingredients together. Turn on to a floured board, and roll the pastry into a long strip. Fold it in three, and press the edges together. Half turn the pastry, rib it with the rolling pin to equalize the air in it, and again roll it into a strip. Fold in three and repeat this until the pastry has had four rolls, folds and half-turns. It is then ready for use.

Sweetening

Sugar

We are all getting sweeter by the decade. About 30% sweeter since the 1980's, making an annual consumption of 160 pounds!

The effects of sugars are causing disease to the old and young alike, diabetes is at an all time high! Sugar is in almost everything, even where we don't expect it or don't want it, like in salty foods and toothpaste. Biologically, as cave dwellers, we needed to sample the surrounding vegetation to check its sweetness and therefore it's safeness to eat. Sweet is safe. Or so we think. What we think of as not being sweet, actually is, but our sweet receptors are in so inundated with sweetness that we can not detect true or natural levels of sweetness. For example, red peppers are sweet, but only to the few that seriously avoid sugar.

One in three North Americans have a weight problem and one in eight New Yorkers have diabetes. This should not be considered acceptable. A typical breakfast of cereal is loaded with sugar and some with chocolate. Our blood sugar levels spike and our pancreas needs to correct it, which is it's job. Only for us to knowingly or unknowingly, cause more spikes later during the day. The pancreas does a very good job, for decades, but like any other organ that is subjected to misuse, it may become problematic.

Sugar has replaced nutrients in our daily diets. Creating all sorts of serious health consequences: obesity, diabetes, heart problems, tooth decay, depletion of limited nutrients, suppressing the immune system, corrupting the body's mineral balance, hyperactivity, anxiety, concentration difficulties, crankiness, drowsiness, weakens defences against bacterial infections, kidney damage, reduces HDL's, raises cholesterol, trace mineral depletion, weakened eyesight, narrow blood vessels, hypoglycemia, acidic stomach, and raises your body's PH levels creating the perfect host environment for cancer.

I use raw (organic) sugar for about half of my sugar uses, Stevia and honey for the other half. This type of sugar is available at any health food store and comes in varying shades. The darker the sugar, the more brown sugar-like it will taste, which isn't always what we want. A pale tan sugar still retains some of it's trace minerals yet won't add a brown sugar taste to your drinks and foods.

If you do have problems with blood sugar levels, you may wish to avoid any type of sugar entirely. Please read on for information about Stevia.

Stevia

Stevia is a naturally sweet, herbal plant. Native to South America, it has been used for centuries by the Guarani Indians of Paraguay as a sweetener for herbal teas and other beverages. Today it is cultivated in Mexico, Paraguay, Central America, Japan, China, Malaysia, South Korea and very recently, Canada.

The measurement of sweetness is a technical matter which is defined precisely. Dried stevia leaves are 30 to 40 times as sweet as sucrose. When the steviosides (the sweet compounds) are extracted from stevia leaves and then isolated and purified, the result can be 250 to 300 times as sweet as sucrose. One should not jump to the conclusion that stevia is "equal" to a certain amount of sugar. In wanting to create recipes using stevia, you may need to run a few experiments to get the right quantities. Also, stevia contains of many phytonutrients not found in sugar: chromium, manganese, selenium, silicon, iron, niacin, phosphorus, potassium, riboflavin, thiamine, Vitamin C, bioflavonoids and zinc. The body may be able to assimilate these trace nutrients more easily in their stevia form that from other sources.

Current research shows that Stevia is anti-viral, anti-bacterial, anti-fungal, and antiseptic, making it beneficial for use in shampoos and oral surgery. Blood sugar control using stevia may help in diabetes, hypoglycemia, hyperactivity, and attention deficit disorder. Stevia has been used in South America to treat hypoglycemia, gingivitis and candida.

Soda Pop manufacturers are just waiting for the green light in order to start promoting their all natural (presumably) and zero calorie drinks. Use this great plant for all your sweetening needs without the calories of real sugar or the chemicals of synthetic sweeteners.

Although the FDA is stalling on the allowing of Stevia to be considered a food additive, Japan has been using Stevia for 30 years with no reported ill effects. Unlike artificial sweeteners that cause numerous ill effects that are all well documented.

The Stevia leaf contain trace minerals and phytonutrients and is much sweeter than sugar. I use Stevia to create all natural and sweet drinks such as Iced Tea and Lemonade.

Stevia also has no carbohydrates, causes no tooth decay and is diabetic safe. It also does not raise blood glucose levels and with no calories and no carbs, it is a great weight loss aid. Stevia is reported to minimize hunger sensations, reduce craving for sweet or fatty foods, aid in digestion, decrease hypertension, stabilize blood glucose levels, and has antibacterial properties when added to toothpastes or mouthwashes. Dr. Mowrey sums it up with this report: "More elaborate safety tests were performed by the Japanese during their evaluation of Stevia as a possible sweetening agent. Few substances have ever yielded such consistently negative results in toxicity trial as have Stevia. Almost every toxicity test imaginable has been performed on Stevia extract (concentrate) or stevioside at one time or another. The results are always negative. No abnormalities in weight change, food intake, cell or membrane characteristics, enzyme and substrate utilization, or chromosome characteristics. No cancer, no birth defects, no acute and no chronic untoward effects. Nothing."

A member of the chrysanthemum family (closely related to tarragon and chamomile and distantly related to lettuce, artichokes, safflower oil, and sunflower seeds and oil), it is totally safe and has been used for centuries by the natives of South America where it grows wild. An interesting contrast: while no one in Japan has complained about any Stevia related health problems for the past thirty years, over 75% of food additive related complaints in the US are about Aspartame, which is supposedly safe.

Honey

Honey was the sweetener of choice to the Celts, although some cane sugar could be obtained through the long and involved shipping process, honey was easier. Nectar, obtained by the honey bees, is composed of mainly sucrose and water. Bees add enzymes, altering the sucrose into fructose and glucose, the water is mostly evaporated, leaving a honey that will now resist spoiling. Honey is 80% natural sugar and sweeter than table sugar; 18% water (a little remains) and 2% minerals, vitamins pollen and protein. The vitamins present are B6, thiamine, niacin, riboflavin, pantothenic acid and amino acids. The minerals found are calcium, copper, iron, magnesium, manganese, phosphorus, potassium, sodium and zinc.

Honey also carries antioxidants, is fat free, cholesterol free, and sodium free.

Honey contains 64 calories per tablespoon, which is more than sugar, but less is needed. The Glycemic Index of honey is 55, sugar is 61. Honey is gradually absorbed into the bloodstream and result in better digestion and a lower GI index.

Give honey a chance, I use in herbal teas as a sweetener, as well as in my Iced Tea (melt the honey with hot water first). Hot Honey and Lemon can be used an appetite suppressant, as well as medicinally for sore throats. Children under one still cannot have honey due to the natural occurring spores that have no effect on those older.

Synthetics

What one could write about synthetic or artificial sweeteners could fill text after text. Study after study has concluded that these sugar mimicking chemicals are not in your best interest to consume. Japan has banned artificial sweeteners for the past 30 years.

These chemicals come in very benign names such as NutraSweet, Equal, Sweet N' Low, and less creative names such as aspartame, acesulfame potassium, sucralose, neotame, and cyclamate. It's true name, it's chemical composition name is 'L-aspartyl-Lphenylalanyl-methyl ester'. Corporations that have created these sweet tasting chemicals in their laboratories, consider this chemical to be safe. Yet every other research team that is not associated with these particular companies, find this chemical not safe. I myself, have in the past, drank Diet Coke, and shortly thereafter feeling a pressure in my head. Look up aspartame on the internet, you'll be wondering why this chemical has not been banned from the shelf.

Barley and Rye Barley

Contains eight essential amino acids, and eating whole grain barley can regulate blood sugar for up to 10 hours after consumption compared to white or even whole-grain wheat, which has a similar glycemic index. The effect was attributed to colonic fermentation of indigestible carbohydrates. Barley can also be used as a coffee substitute.

Hulled barley (or covered barley) is eaten after removing the inedible, fibrous outer hull. Once removed, it is called dehulled barley (or pot barley or scotch barley) and considered a whole grain. Dehulled barley still has its bran and germ making it a nutritious and popular health food. Pearl barley (or pearled barley) is dehulled barley which has been steam processed further to remove the bran. It may be polished, a process known as pearling. Dehulled or pearl barley may be processed into a variety of barley products, including flour, flakes similar to oatmeal, and grits.

Barley-meal, a wholemeal barley flour, is lighter than wheatmeal but darker in color, is used in porridge and gruel in old Celtic times. The six row variety *bere* is cultivated in Orkney, Shetland, Caithness and the Western Isles in the Scottish Highlands and islands. The grain is used to make *beremeal*, used locally in bread, biscuits, and the traditional *beremeal bannock*.

The nutritional facts of barley are Vitamins B1, B2, B3, B5, B6, B9, C, Calcium, Iron, Magnesium, Phosphorus, Potassium and Zinc.

Rye

Barley Rye bread, including pumpernickel, is a widely eaten food in Northern and Eastern Europe. Rye is also used to make the familiar crisp bread. Rye flour has a lower gluten content than wheat flour, and contains a higher proportion of soluble fiber.

Other uses of rye include rye whiskey and an alternative medicine known as rye extract. Rye straw is used to make corn dollies.

In medieval Europe, bread made from barley and rye was peasant food, while wheat products were consumed by the upper classes. Potatoes largely replaced barley in Eastern Europe in the 19th century.

Contemporary Additions

We can add some great last-century additions to our diet and health plans to create what is going to be the perfect health and weight loss plan today. The first part of this chapter details some of the best items to incorporate into your daily routine. The second part tells us of some of the things we really need to avoid in order to gain our health and fitness back.

Green tea

For centuries, green tea has held strong to its reputation as a very effective and trustworthy anti-oxidant, and the Chinese have been using it for over 4,000 years to treat problems like headaches. The benefits of drinking this tea include providing preventative measures to deter diseases and other problems such as high cholesterol, cleansing and removing toxins from the body.

Green tea contains certain vitamins in which it is particularly rich in EGCG or epigallocatechil gallate. This is a powerful anti-oxidant that has an effect against cancer cell growth without harming the rest of the healthy tissues in the body.

The production of green tea and many other kinds of tea originated from China. Black tea, jasmine tea, and all the other types do have their own healing properties, giving similar benefits in the body. But Green tea and all the other teas manufactured differ in their processes. Green tea leaves are steamed, which prevents the epigallocatechil gallate from becoming oxidized unlike the black tea and the oolong tea leaves, which are fermented and are converted into compounds that are not as effective in preventing and fighting diseases and illnesses as green tea.

Green tea is natural, so you can expect very few side effects, or maybe none, when drinking it regularly. Other benefits that have been discovered recently include effective burning of calories when mixed with caffeine, and the prevention of tooth decay and food poisoning because of its ability to destroy bacteria as well.

Even products for the exterior such as the skin care contain green tea.

Green Tea is great with a little lemon juice. Try adding a bag of green tea to the ground coffee in your coffee maker, we well as adding a bag of green tea to two orange pekoe tea bags when making Iced Tea.

Coffee

It's the rich aroma, robust flavor, increased energy and alertness that are appreciated by coffee lovers. But now, medical studies are adding the prevention of cancer, liver disease and a number of other serious illnesses to that list.

Coffee got bad attention previously for its high caffeine content and possible side effects. But the health benefits associated with coffee can still be obtained with a moderate daily coffee intake. Many components of coffee act as natural shields against the development of these conditions. For instance, caffeine is known to help prevent liver cancer, and the many antioxidants found in coffee reduce the chances of developing cancer. Antioxidants of all types are widely believed to protect cells and tissues in our bodies from oxidative damage. Oxidative damage to these cells often results in the development of cancerous cells. Antioxidants are also known to help prevent heart disease—another major killer.

These two antioxidants found in coffee beans are caffeic acid and chlorogenic acid. The oil in the coffee beans also contains anti-carcinogenic agents, further helping to reduce the chances of developing cancer. The only negative about coffee and disease is that coffee may reduce the output of bile acids which may play a role in allowing disease, like cancer, in the colon.

In the past, caffeine was on the 'bad' list for diabetics, as the caffeine could elevate heart rate, which could release adrenaline, that would release stored sugars into the blood stream and thus affect diabetic symptoms. Now, the prevention of Type 2 diabetes, (the most common form of the disease) is also among the new found benefits of drinking coffee. A number of tests conducted in the US over the past decade have shown that regular coffee drinking can reduce the risk of developing diabetes by as much as 50 percent. Considering that 150 million people worldwide are suffering from Type 2 these results are crucial.

Another well-known and severely debilitating condition that coffee can help prevent is Parkinson's Disease. Studies have shown that people who drink at least four cups of coffee a day are five times less likely to develop Parkinson's Disease due to coffee's high caffeine content. Some of the more common and temporary benefits of drinking coffee is caffeine's rapid effect on headaches and preventing and treating asthma attacks.

It is suggested that to gain the above benefits of drinking coffee is to consume three to five cups a day. If you do have a problem with caffeine, consider half-decaffeinated versions or mix your own special blend of half and half.

Psyllium

Plantago ovata is a plant that is primarily grown in Iran and India and contains stalks that have seeds, which are called psyllium, and used in Indian culture for hundreds of years. The seeds are covered in a husk which forms a gel like substance containing mucilage, that finds its way into foods to add fiber, especially breakfast cereals. The United States is one of the largest importers of psyllium, as high as 60%, and mucilages are found in products, such as Metamucil.

Psyllium fiber is not broken down as it passes through the system and has no other nutritional value besides being a source of fiber. By adding water to psyllium fiber, it swells to ten times its original size, so it finds its way into a lot of weight loss products and plans. The combination of a low fat diet, low in saturated fats and cholesterol plus the addition of psyllium can reduce cholesterol due to reduced absorption by the intestines. It has also been found that psyllium fiber incorporated into food products is effective at lowering levels of blood glucose.

The benefits of taking psyllium fiber to promote weight loss, would come through its ability to enable digestion without much absorption, much like a cleanse agent, and its ability to swell up with water. Besides making you feel fuller, a healthy digestive system eliminates excess fat and toxins. Because 1 tablespoon equals a bowl of bran cereal, by adding 1-3 tablespoons to your daily diet, it satisfies appetite cravings, which cause you to feel full for longer. It is best to start off by taking 1 tablespoon a day for the first week and gradually add up to the 3 tablespoons per day.

Another benefit of aiding in weight loss is that it comes in an odorless and tasteless powder form, so it can be added to foods to increase the fiber and of feeling full. It also comes in pill form, which can be taken about 30 minutes before a meal, but powder form can just be sprinkled on food, or added to a smoothie or protein shake to make it thicker. Many dieters add a little to anything they have, so they get psyllium fiber in smaller, regular doses, instead of all at once.

It has been recommended by numerous health professionals and is available at most health food stores. The possible side effects could be gas since it is a natural laxative. So monitor your dosage carefully for the first few days as your system gets used to it.

By adding psyllium fiber to your diet, not only will you feel more satisfied and eat less if you are dieting, it acts as a natural colon cleanse, and is good for heart disease, diabetes, high triglycerides, and irritable bowel syndrome. The benefits of taking psyllium fiber to promote weight loss, may have other benefits, as well.

I would suggest the powder form and add to your foods. I have tried the husks and they seem 'crunchy' when you eat or drink them. Another thought about this amazing fibre is that it does taste a little like dried grass clippings, so I'd suggest adding it to juice or what have you. Make sure to follow your initial psyllium drink with a glass of water, the fibre will need water in order to expand properly. And the longer it sits in your glass the thicker it gets, so drink quickly.

Try adding psyllium to a breakfast cereal, a fruit smoothie, into yogurt, add to your baking, shake the powder on salads, casseroles or stew, replace a little of the bread crumbs in meat loaf.

Water

Water is not really a contemporary addition, but in a way it is. We have been drinking liquids that are sweet and foamy, or tart and colorful, and going back to plain water may seem boring. There are numerous books out there talking about the benefits of plain water. Here we will talk about the well known benefits and some of the lesser known ones.

The human body is comprised of more than seventy percent water, and we are not born with the amount of water we need for a lifetime. Our bodies use water every second to keep us running, and when it gets used, it must be replaced. From our head to our toes, we need water everywhere for everything. When muscles are used, they are losing water. When we breathe we use between two and four cups of water every day. Ordinary everyday perspiration can use up another two cups of water. Urinating uses even more.

Every cell needs water to work properly, it helps the cells to process blood, which is also mostly water. Organs and joints tend to work better when supplied with adequate water. Not only does water lubricate, but it hydrates as well to promote proper flow throughout all organs and body systems. Muscle discomfort can be reduced with plenty of water as well.

The benefits of drinking water can be seen superficially as well, on our skin. Our skin is probably the most obviously benefited recipient of adequate hydration. Skin looks younger and wrinkles are visibly reduced with adequate water consumption.

It does seem difficult to drink plain water all day when we are used to flavored water, be it cola or coffee or juice. Choose the right temperature of water that suits you best. Perhaps cold water is just too cold unless it is summer and hot. Have a jug of water on the counter, at room temperature, which could be easier to drink. And room temperature doesn't mean that it is warm, because the water is at 70 degrees and we are at 98.6 degrees, so the water is a perfect cool temperature when drinking. Adding a shot of lemon juice helps immensely.

Water is important to the digestive system. It can help to digest food better as well as reduce the occurrence of constipation. Drinking lots of water can also decreased bloating. The body processes and flushes out unwanted waste matter using just water.

There are more reasons as well. People who drink enough water every day are less likely to experience depression and irritability. Blood pressure and body temperature can also benefit positively from water.

Some people claim a cup of warm water can also be very calming right before bed. Others claim that shedding unwanted weight is more successful when drinking hot water.

Exercise

The Celts were only too familiar with exercise, although to them it was just the way it was. From before sunrise to after sunset. We are talking about activities such as field work, sword fighting, cutting peat bogs, gardening, stable work, walking absolutely everywhere or riding a horse, hunting, hauling water, house/barn/stable building, ploughing, planting, picking fruits and vegetables, storing and preserving the same, cutting firewood, making all clothes by recycling fabrics and hand stitching, making dishes out of wood, hauling rocks and making fireplaces, tending to other farm animals, making every meal from scratch, washing clothes by hand, and . . . well, you get the picture.

So how to replace all this physical activity? And do it as simply as you can to ensure success. Devise a method that is going to work for you, and this could be a way that is done by no one else. So far I have heard routines consisting of dancing to favorite songs, using the elliptical while watching favorite tv shows on dvd (1 hour shows are 40 minutes with no commercials!), rebounding, walking around the nearby cemetery (it's level and nearby), going to the gym at really early hours (5 am-630 am is quieter), walking around the house while on the phone, reading novels while on the treadmill, exercising on the bed because the floor is too hard. Get an exercise DVD and follow that. Check YouTube, there are a lot of free exercise routines that you can try. Try a different one every week. Think about what you don't like about trying to exercise think of some way to avoid that pitfall.

Vitamins

Some health professionals once thought that you don't need supplements if you eat right. That is easier said than done, especially when our foods are grown under duress from being genetically modified, sprayed with numerous chemicals, and in nutrient depleted soils.

While eating better can prevent much disease, doctors and scientists finally recognize that supplements play a very important role. Our bodies require 40 essential micronutrients, including vitamins, minerals and other bionutrients. All of which are almost impossible to obtain from our diets. It is estimated that millions of cases of heart disease, cancer, strokes and birth defects could have been prevented with a simple multivitamin.

In short, vitamins are essential to good health. Vitamin A helps to develop and maintain body tissues such as bone and skin; it also helps the body's vision, nervous system functioning, reproduction, and growth. The B vitamins are responsible for increasing the production of fats, proteins, and carbohydrates as well as assisting with metabolism, building red blood cells, and maintaining the protective covering of the nervous system.

Vitamin C helps form tissues, cells, bones and teeth; heals wounds; and improves the immune system's performance. Vitamin E protects the outer cell membranes from harm, thus assisting the immune system in fighting off diseases. Vitamin K helps the body's blood clot in wounded areas.

Also, there are the minerals, that also have a broad range of functions. As many as 20 minerals play significant roles in the body. "Microminerals," or "trace minerals", are minerals that the body only needs traces of in order to fight off serious illness. These include copper, iodine, chromium, iron, fluorine, tin, zinc, nickel, vanadium, manganese, silicon, molybdenum, and selenium. Minerals that the body needs larger amounts of include magnesium, sodium, potassium, chlorine, phosphorus, calcium, and sulfur.

Zinc is responsible for helping metabolize proteins and keeping enzymes functioning. Copper is needed by enzymes for metabolizing. Iodine assists the thyroid gland in working properly. Calcium and phosphorus build bones and teeth. Iron delivers oxygen to the body's cells. Potassium helps muscle contraction, maintains the fluid balance of cells, helps transmit messages through the body's nerves, and keeps the kidneys and heart working correctly.

Vitamins and minerals not only help the body function, but they work to strengthen each other. The body absorbs iron through the help of vitamin C. Vitamin D helps the body absorb phosphorus and calcium. Vitamins D and K are the only vitamins the body can supply for itself. The skin creates vitamin D when it is exposed to sunlight. Vitamin K is produced by intestinal bacteria. Outside sources must supply the body with all other vitamins.

Vitamins are divided into two categories, namely by the substance that carries them throughout the body. Water-soluble vitamins are carried and stored all throughout the body by water. These vitamins need daily replacement because they are lost in body fluids such as sweat and urine. Water-soluble vitamins include folacin (folic acid), biotin, pantothenic acid, thiamin (B1), riboflavin (B2), niacin (B3), pyridoxine (B6), and cyanocobalamin (B12). Fat-soluble vitamins—these vitamins, such as A (retinol), D (calciferol), E (d-alpha-tocopherol), and K (menaquinone), are carried by fats located in the bloodstream. Since fat stores better than water, it is less critical when the intake of these vitamins is interrupted than when water-soluble vitamin intake is interrupted. However, when extreme amounts of these vitamins are taken, toxic levels can become present in the body.

Already, Americans spend over 6 billion dollars annually on vitamins. A poll in 1998 that showed 71% of Americans take at least one form of vitamin or mineral supplementation.

Most people do not eat ideal diets. According to a national survey, over half of all Americans do not drink a glass of juice, eat one serving of vegetables, or eat a piece of fruit daily. Only 40% eat 3 to 5 servings of vegetables daily, the recommended amount. Only 20% eat the recommend 2 to 4 servings of fruit each day. For those not eating properly, supplementation is better than nothing.

We all have read or heard about how in third world countries, or from our history books, that even small amounts of vitamins or minerals missing from our daily foods can cause harm. You know yourself and your diet. There are numerous reasons as to why some people may be lacking particular nutrients, for example, vegetarians tend to lack the required amount of iron needed as meat sources provide the most easily absorbable iron.

Fresh air

People are spending more time than ever inside. In fact, in 2006 the average employed person spent 7.6 hours at work on a working day, then another 2.5 to 3 hours watching TV. That's over 10 hours of indoor time right there, and that doesn't include the time you're asleep. If you sleep for seven hours a night, that's at least 17 hours of indoor time every day.

Meanwhile, the numbers of visitors to the country's national parks are falling. And, according to other statistics, every week kids are spending seven hours more on academics, and two hours less on sports and outdoor activities, than they did two decades ago. Getting fresh air is great for your body and mind, while indoor air is quite possibly hazardous for your health.

According to the U.S. Environmental Protection Agency (EPA), who states:

"In the last several years, a growing body of scientific evidence has indicated that the air within homes and other buildings can be more seriously polluted than the outdoor air in even the largest and most industrialized cities. Other research indicates that people spend approximately 90 percent of their time indoors. Thus, for many people, the risks to health may be greater due to exposure to air pollution indoors than outdoors."

And what is in your indoor air at home? It's chlorine gas from your cleaning products, pieces of cockroaches and other bugs, microscopic dust mites, molds and fungus.

Meanwhile, at work, a cubic meter of air in your office contains several hundred fungal spores, 89 micrograms of ethanol, 42 micrograms of acetone, 16 micrograms of formaldehyde, 1/2 microgram of chloroform, byproducts of your coworkers' such as flatulence and skin cells.

While outdoor air isn't always perfect either, you can do your body (and your mind) good by making it a point to get some fresh air everyday. So when weather permits, read that book outside, take that walk, sit on the balcony. Even small doses of fresh air help reap benefits.

For those of you can't always be outside, and need to improve on the air inside, there are some helpful solutions. Purifying your indoor air using air filtering and purifying devices that use photocatalysis, which is designed to oxidize organic odors, germs, and fungi. This technology creates ultraviolet light rays, safe levels of ozone, and passive negative ions as part of your air treatment.

Simply cleaning can reduce a significant amount of toxins in your indoor air from dirt and dust that, through everyday living, end up on almost every surface in your home. Cleaning these surfaces is therefore necessary to reduce the toxins in your air, as when you walk around you stir up that dirt and dust into the air you breathe.

Using doormats, this allows up to 90% of tracked in dirt and toxins to be left in a mat that captures this debris instead of letting it be tracked throughout the home. Have a doormat on the outside to wipe shoes on and one on the inside to catch the rest.

Organic, not processed

The debate will continue forever on whether Organic produce or products are better than the conventionally grown produce. Yet we can't avoid the logic that if chemicals are on our food, and these particular chemicals are toxic, then they are going to cause some damage. As genetically grown produce takes over the farming community, our food is not what it used to be. The same food that our entire human race is comprised of. Our bodies are created to utilize all the natural nutrients in food, and this has been going on since the beginning of time. The GM crops contain components that we would not eat if given the choice.

The Biochemical Institute at the University of Texas, Austin states the average vegetable found in today's supermarket is anywhere from 5% to 40% lower in minerals (including magnesium, iron, calcium and zinc) than those harvested just 50 years ago. A review of 41 studies comparing the nutritional value of organically to conventionally grown fruits, vegetables and grains, also indicates organic crops provide substantially more of several nutrients, including:

-60% more disease fighting phenols than traditionally farmed produce. In a study, corn grown with little or no pesticides had almost 60 percent higher levels of phenols than conventionally grown corn. Strawberries were nearly 20 percent higher in phenols;

-27% more vitamin C;

-21.1% more iron;

-29.3% more magnesium;

-13.6% more phosphorus.

-researchers suspect that pesticide use somehow inhibits the formation of these nutrients.

In all industrialized countries, it can be assumed that just about all tap drinking water contains pesticide residues and with the exception of organic foods, so does the food supply.

Even small doses of pesticides and other chemicals can adversely affect people, especially during vulnerable periods of fetal development and childhood when exposures can have long lasting effects. The negative impact of pesticides on our health, even at very small trace levels, is well documented. Pesticide exposure compromises the liver's ability to process other toxins, the cells' ability to produce energy, and the nerves' ability to send messages. Because the toxic effects of pesticides are worrisome, not well understood, or in some cases completely unstudied, shoppers are wise to minimize exposure to pesticides whenever possible.

While in your grocery store, check the prices or organic produce, you may find it comparable, and even less than conventional if on sale.

Contemporary additions to AVOID

Below are not-so-friendly contemporary additions to our food supply that we are going to attempt to avoid. The giant food corporations and conglomerations have one criteria, and that is to sell more food and beverage products to consumers. These food companies are not "food companies" exactly, they are businesses with a bottom line and that line is to be successful and increase profits to themselves and their stockholders. Their aim is not to improve your health or help you in any way. Their aim is to create a product that you will buy. Period. And this type of success is paramount to you being kept in the dark about certain issues such as the presence cancer-causing chemicals found in popular food products.

Here are ten things the food corporations, whose products dominate grocery store shelves across the United States and other countries, absolutely do not want you to know.

1. The ingredients listed on the label aren't the only things in the food. Cancer-causing chemicals such as **acrylamides** may be formed in the food during high-heat processing, yet there's no requirement to list them on the label. Residues of solvents, pesticides and other chemicals may also be present, but also do not have to be listed. The National Uniformity for Food Act, currently being debated in the U.S. Congress, would make it illegal (yes, illegal) for states to require cancer warnings on foods that contain cancer-causing chemicals (such as California's Proposition 65).

2. **Monosodium glutamate** (MSG), which is added to thousands of food and grocery products through a dozen different innocent-sounding names, imbalances endocrine system function, disabling normal appetite regulation and causing consumers to keep eating more food. This chemical not only contributes to nationwide obesity, it also helps food companies boost repeat business. MSG is routinely hidden in foods by using these FDA approved names: yeast extract, torula yeast, hydrolyzed vegetable protein and autolyzed yeast. Thousands of common grocery products contain one or more of these chemical taste enhancers, including "vegetarian" foods such as veggie burgers.

3. **Natural or organic** anything. The organized, yet not enforceable, usage of the words natural and organic have led to a serious misleading to consumers. Take 'naturally inspired' for example, if we remember our grade 5 language

studies, the word 'naturally' is actually describing the word 'inspired', not the product itself. And the word 'organic' really means that something has a carbon molecule. Period. Which means that we are organic.

4. **Artificial colors** and refined carbohydrates are being recognized as being the leading cause of ADHD in children. Eighty percent of alleged ADHD children who are taken off processed foods are miraculously cured of ADHD in two weeks. If we were to see some of our food without these colors, we would want to know what was wrong with them.

5. The chemical sweetener **aspartame,** when exposed to warm temperatures for only a few hours, begins to break down into chemicals like formaldehyde and formic acid. Formaldehyde is a potent nerve toxin and causes damage to the eyes, brain and entire nervous system. Aspartame has been strongly linked to migraines, seizures, blurred vision and many other nervous system problems. I personally know that this ingredient causes headaches.

6. Most **food dips** (like guacamole dip) are made with hydrogenated oils, artificial colors and monosodium glutamate. Many guacamole dips don't even contain avocados.

7. **Plastic food packaging** is a potent health hazard. Scientists now know that plastics routinely seep the chemical bisphenol A into the food, where it is eaten by consumers. Cooking in plastic containers multiplies the level of exposure. Bisphenol is a hormone disruptor and can cause breast formation in men and severe hormonal imbalances in women. It may also encourage hormone-related cancers such as prostate cancer and breast cancer.

8. **Milk** produced in the United States comes from cows injected with synthetic hormones that have been banned in every other advanced nation in the world. These hormones help explain why young girls develop breasts and start their menstration as early as 6 years old. Or why hormone-related cancers like prostate cancer are being discovered in unprecedented numbers. In order to protect Monsanto (the manufacturer of hormones used in the industry) the USDA currently bans organic milk producers from claiming their milk comes from cows that were not treated with synthetic hormones. Even organic milk is now under fire as the Organic Consumers Association says Horizon milk products are falsely labeled

as organic. If these synthetic hormones can bulk up a cow, they can certainly bulk you up. Your options here are, raw almond milk, rice milk, soy milk, or milk and dairy products produced and imported from Canada, where these hormones are banned.

9. Most grocery products that make loud **health claims** on their packaging are, in reality, nutritionally worthless. Packaging claims such as "health check" and "vitamin enriched" mean virtually nothing. Perhaps there is fibre in this product (like cereals) and maybe there are vitamins added, this does not mean that this product is actually healthy for you. It simply means that there is fibre and vitamins, the benefits of which are no doubt eliminated by the 98% of unhealthy ingredients. The most nutritious foods are actually those the FDA does not allow to make any health claims whatsoever, like fresh produce.

10. Food manufacturers actually **"buy" shelf space** and position at grocery stores. That's why the most profitable foods and coincidentally, the ones with the lowest quality ingredients, are the most visible on aisle end caps, checkout lanes and eye-level shelves throughout the store. The effect of all this is to provide in-store marketing and visibility to the very foods and beverages that promote obesity, diabetes, cancer, heart disease and other degenerative conditions now ravaging consumers around the world.

The Oats

It is in this chapter that we learn about the one critical ingredient that is going to put us on the right track to a healthy diet and healthy lifestyle. It is as simple as oatmeal. The Celtic Nations were a healthy, resourceful, ready to fight or flight, and oats contributed to that.

80% of North Americans already have oats or oatmeal in their kitchen. This simple and inexpensive grain is about to bring you much deserved health benefits that you deserve. Let's start with the different types of oatmeal available, although they all start from the same oats.

Oat groats are the unflattened kernels that are good for using as a cereal or for stuffing.

Steel Cut oats are whole oat groats that have been chopped into about three smaller pieces. This type of oatmeal is usually preferred although it takes a little longer to cook than it's instant counterparts. With Steel Cut oats, the oatmeal is creamy and the oats chewy.

Rolled oats are the oat groats that have been steamed rolled and flaked for easier cooking.

Quick cooking oats are rolled oats that have been chopped into smaller pieces. These take more time than the powdered instant variety, yet less time than the uncut rolled oats.

Instant Oats are basically powdered oats. This type of oat doesn't always produce a great bowl of oatmeal, creating more of a paste. Although very good for other purposes that you will read about here.

Oat Bran is the outer layer of the grain that is located under the hull. The oat bran is usually still contained in the rolled and steel-cut oats, it can also be bought as a separate products.

Oat flour is used in baking, often combined with wheat or other gluten-containing flours, to make breads.

Oats, known scientifically as Avena sativa, are a hardy cereal grain able to grow in poor soil conditions in which other crops are unable to thrive. Oats gain part of their distinctive flavor from the roasting process that they undergo after being harvested and cleaned. Although oats are then hulled, this process does not strip away their bran and germ allowing them to retain a concentrated source of their fiber and nutrients.

Oatmeal is not just for breakfast anymore. It deserves more of a limelight in our everyday food consumption. Let's read about its numerous benefits.

Lowering Cholesterol Levels with beta-glucan, a specific type of fiber contained in the oats, oat bran and oatmeal. Study after study, since 1963, has proven the effects of this fiber on cholesterol levels. For those with high cholesterol (above 220 mg/dl), a small consumption of 3 grams of soluble oat fiber per day (one bowlful) lowers cholesterol by 8-23%. For every 1% drop in serum cholesterol equates a 2% drop in the risk of developing heart disease. High cholesterol equals plaques building up in the blood vessels, which can equal a blockage or vessel rupture and causing a heart attack, stroke, or blood clot. Lowering cholesterol can avoid these serious health risks.

A Unique Oat Antioxidant called avenanthramides, also reduce the risk of cardiovascular disease by preventing free radicals from damaging LDL cholesterol equaling a reduction in heart disease.

Whole grains and heart failure prevention. Drug treatment for heart failure remains poor, statins have not been found safe or effective. Of 2445 discharged heart failure patients, 37.3 percent died the first year and 78.5% died within 5 years.

A very long study of (non refined) cereal for breakfast eaters over 19 years found that there was a 29% lower risk of heart failure. That is a significant number.

Postmenopausal women with high cholesterol, high blood pressure or other signs of heart disease are increasing their health benefits with at least 6 servings of whole grains such as oats. Studies have showed the reduced risk of built up plague in the vessel walls as well as less narrowing of arterial passageways. Interestingly, fiber from fruits and vegetables alone did not match the heart disease risk reduction when whole grains were added.

Beta-glucan again still has more benefits, that being the ability to **Enhance Immune Response** to Infection. Laboratory studies show beta-glucan assists the immune system in responding to bacterial infections. Both in getting to the infection site more quickly and an increased ability to eliminate the bacteria found.

Stabilize Blood Sugar, and with the Type 2 Diabetes epidemic in North America today, we need natural stabilizers to help us to control this disease. Studies have indicated that diabetics who were given foods high in oat fiber or oatmeal, experienced much lower rises in their blood sugar levels, compared with those given white rice or bread. Starting your day with a blood sugar stabilizer as oatmeal makes it easier to keep blood sugar levels under control for the rest of the day.

And if you don't have diabetes yet, or there is a family disposition, Oats and Other Whole Grains **Substantially Lower Type 2 Diabetes Risk.** Magnesium is a mineral that acts as a co-factor for over 300 enzymes that are needed in the body for glucose and insulin secretion. And Oats and other whole grains are a rich source for this mineral.

A large study of women's eating habits showed that those women who ate oats or whole grains had a 31% lower risk of diabetes. Yet in the same study where woman consumed magnesium as a supplement, there was still a substantial but lower rate of 19% in the risk of diabetes. This outcome implying that the whole grains alone decreased the risk of diabetes by another 39% over magnesium supplements alone.

More Antioxidant Benefits with selenium are also realized in oats. Selenium is a cofactor of the important antioxidant glutathione peroxidase, working with vitamin E and numerous vital systems throughout the body. Selenium helps in decreasing asthma symptoms and preventing heart disease. Selenium is also involved in the repair of DNA and the decreased risk of cancers.

Breast Cancer too is significantly reduced, by half, in premenopausal woman who eat approximately 30 grams of fiber per day. That is a 52% lower risk of breast cancer compared to women whose diets supplied the least fiber, being 20 grams per day.

Whole grains, now found to be equal to vegetable and fruits. The powerful phytonutrients in oats and whole grains have largely been unrecognized because of the research methods used to detect them. Previously, phytonutrients were measured in their free-form being absorbed into the bloodstream. The whole grains bound-form are released during digestion before they are absorbed.

One major class of phytonutrients is the powerful antioxidant phenolics. When the free-form and the bound form of phenolics where being measured in common fruits and vegetables, the average number of free-forms were 76%. In whole grains, the free-form was 1% and the bound-forms were a whopping 99%. Until the adaptable measuring system had been initiated, the measure benefits of whole grains have been greatly underestimated.

Despite the differences in fruits, vegetables and whole grains content of free-and bound-formed phenolics, the total antioxidant activity in all three types of whole foods is similar. Testing the antioxidant activity of various foods, assigning each a rating based on a formula of vitamin C per gram, broccoli and spinach measured 80 and 81; apple and banana measured 98 and 65; whole wheat 77, oats 75, and brown rice 56.

This explains why studies have shown that populations eating diets high in fiber-rich whole grains consistently have lower risk for colon cancer, yet short-term clinical trials that have focused on fiber alone in lowering colon cancer risk, often to the point of giving subjects isolated fiber supplements, yield inconsistent results. The explanation is most likely that these studies have not taken into account the interactive effects of all the nutrients in whole grains—not just their fiber, but also their many phytonutrients.

It is believed that the key to their powerful cancer-fighting potential is precisely their wholeness. A grain of whole wheat consists of three parts-its endosperm (starch), bran and germ. When wheat-or any whole grain-is refined, its bran and germ are removed. Although these two parts make up only 15-17% of the grain's weight, they contain 83% of its phenolics. Recent findings on the antioxidant content of whole grains reinforce the message that a variety of foods should be eaten good health. Different plant foods have different phytochemicals, and these substances go to different organs, tissues and cells, where they perform different functions. What your body needs to ward off disease is this synergistic effect—this teamwork—that is produced by eating a wide variety of plant foods, including whole grains like oatmeal.

The typical American diet is laden with foods that, while high in calories, do not make you feel "full." Eating a bowl of healthy oatmeal will make you feel fuller than eating a pint of ice cream, but that single bowl of oatmeal nevertheless provides you with more nutrients and less calories than that entire pint of ice cream. Fiber is the reason behind this apparent paradox. By providing bulk to your diet, fiber fills you up without the extra calories you don't need, making it a natural appetite suppressant.

Six greats ways that oatmeal is going to help you lose weight:

1. It makes you eat slower. It takes most people a lot longer to eat a bowl of oatmeal than a slice of pizza;

2. Since it provides bulk in your intestines, fiber makes you feel "full," so you'll want to eat less. According to a research study reported in Gentle Cures and Natural Medicines, people who drink even just one glass of orange juice with pectin before meals feel fuller and eat less.

3. It stimulates your body to release natural appetite-suppressing hormones like cholecystokinin.

4. By helping your body transport fat and calories through your digestive system, fiber actually increases the amount of calories you excrete in your feces.

5. Soluble fiber, such as psyllium, coats your intestinal tract, reducing the amount of fat your body absorbs. Psyllium does the same job as the OTC diet pill Alli, without the nasty and embarrassing side effects.

6. Soluble fiber slows down your body's release of glucose, so you'll feel hungry less often; this also prevents the onset of type 2 diabetes.

With all these benefits, adding more fiber to your diet just may be one of the most important steps you take to achieve your weight loss goal, maintain a healthy body weight and improve your general health. It's also one of the easiest steps you can take. Health food stores, and even your neighborhood grocery stores, are jam-packed with foods high in soluble and insoluble fiber.

Historically, the modern oat draws its ancestry from the wild red oat, a plant originating in Asia. Oats have been cultivated for two thousand years in various regions throughout the world. Before being consumed as a food, oats were used for medicinal purposes, a use for which they are still honored. The growing of oats in Europe was widespread, and oats constituted an important commercial crop since they were a dietary staple for the people of many countries including Scotland, Great Britain, Germany and the Scandinavian countries. In the early 17th century, Scottish settlers brought oats to North America. Today, the largest commercial producers of oats include the Russian Federation, the United States, Germany, Poland and Finland.

Although oats feel dry, they contain a slightly higher fat content than other grains and may go rancid more quickly. Oats are generally available in prepackaged containers as well as bulk bins. Just as with any other food that you may purchase in the bulk section, make sure that the bins containing the oats are covered, free from debris, and that the store has a good product turnover so as to ensure its maximal freshness. Smell the oats to make sure that they are fresh. Whether purchasing oats in bulk or in a packaged container, make sure there is no evidence of moisture. If you purchase prepared oatmeal products such as oatmeal, look at the ingredients to ensure that the product does not contain any salt, sugar or other additives. Store oatmeal in an airtight container in a cool, dry and dark place where they will keep for approximately two months.

Today, nutritional science has been opening the door for people to start looking at foods that are actually good for them. Its about taking healthy items and putting a new attitude to them, for instance, for those that remember mushy oatmeal, cook up those steel cut oats for a great texture. Old-fashioned was a word that was used to describe oatmeal, and in a world of high technology, old fashioned doesn't seem to make oatmeal desirable, but getting back to nature and eating for health—does.

This healthy eating program and diet plan is going to bring health benefits and a weight loss that is brought about simply by eating simpler. And you can still have dessert!

One of the more important aspects of this plan is that it is **not** going to cost you $100's or $1,000's of dollars. Fact is, this is the only weight loss program that will save you money when shopping.

Cooking these oats is easier than cooking up a traditional breakfast of bacon and eggs or pancakes. You don't have to love cooking in order to make a simple and quick meal of oats. In some respects, the oats can cook themselves. You can soak the oats overnight and heat up in the morning, all because it has absorbed the water it needed without heat.

The Celtic method of breads did not generally include the use of yeast, although baking soda was used when available. Breads were dense and heavy and usually fried or baked on a fire and comprised of a few fairly basic with a few ingredients.

Havercakes or riddlecakes are made from a soft dough or batter, whereas the *sgian* oatcake of the Highland Scots was a firm pastry dough. These cakes/breads are in fact historic as archaeologists have found oatcakes in Iron Age peat bog deposits and havercakes have been mentioned in Langland's Piers Plowman written in the 1300's.

"Too make thin oat Cakes It must bee made with oaten meale steped all night in pump water, and bake it the next morning pore in the batter upon a stove with a brass Ladell."

Baking Soda is pure Sodium Bicarbonate, also called Bicarbonate of Soda ($NaHCO_3$). It is a white crystalline alkali which reacts by effervescing (fizzing) when it comes into contact with acids, thus producing gasses, namely carbon dioxide. Because of this chemical reaction, it is often used in fizzy drinks and antacid remedies and it's precisely this reaction which facilitates the rising action in baked goods. Food historians believe the use of baking soda dates back to ancient civilization and it is perhaps this age-old use of it which has prevented its demise as a chemical additive.

Until the late 1700's, yeast was the main leavening ingredient used. It became widely accepted that bicarbonate of soda would create carbon dioxide gas in the presence of certain acids.

By 1835 the first baking powder compound had been created with the addition of Cream of Tartar. It was found that it gave more consistent results although it was more expensive than bicarbonate of soda and had a shorter shelf life. Experimentation continued and by the 1850s the Cream of Tartar was replaced with calcium phosphate.

However, it wasn't until 1885 when sodium aluminium sulphate was discovered. This acid reacted only when heat was applied. The combination of Bicarbonate of Soda and different acids revolutionized baking powder.

Baking soda was known in ancient civilizations and was one of only two known means of leavening baked goods. (The other was wild yeast.) Irish soda bread is a good example of how baking soda was and is still used for that purpose.

Scottish Oatcakes

Oatcakes are widely considered to be the national bread of Scotland, and have held that position for many centuries. Traditionally, each community had its own mill to grind oats from local crofts and supply oatmeal for every household. These oats formed the Highlanders' staple diet of porridge and oatcakes.

In one history book it is documented that one foreign dignitary commented that in England the oat was given to horses and not to men. To which was responded with, "Which is why England is noted for its horses and Scotland for its men."

North Staffordshire Oatcake

A North Staffordshire oatcake is a type of pancake made from oatmeal, flour and yeast, and cooked on a griddle. These usually have fillings such as cheese, bacon, sausage and egg.

Porridge or *porage*, is a simple dish made by boiling oats, cut or rolled, or another grain meal in water, milk or both. Oat and semolina porridge are in many countries the most popular varieties. Some other grains used for porridge include rice, wheat, peasemeal, barley, and cornmeal. Gruel is a thin porridge made with water.

The differences and varieties are:

-*oatmeal porridge*, can be made with steel-cut oats (traditional in Ireland and Scotland) or with rolled oats (traditional in England and the United States). Known as porridge in the British Isles and as oatmeal in the United States;

-also a traditional Scandinavian and Icelandic breakfast;

-*groats*, a porridge made from unprocessed oats;

-*zacierka*, a polish traditional breakfast made with hot milk, sometimes with sugar and butter;

-*maize porridge*, from cornmeal;

-*grits*, ground hominy, lime cooked cornmeal, traditional in the southern United States;

-*atole*, from corn, popular in Mexico;

-*polenta*, from Italy, cooked cornmeal, often fried too;

-mămăligă, from Romania, thick cooked cornmeal, like a dense bread;

-*atole de chocolate* or *champurrado,* from Spain, cornmeal cooked with sugar, milk, and chocolate;

-ugali, corn flour porridge, from South Africa;

-pease porridge, made from dried peas, traditionally English and Scottish.

Bannock is a bread thinner than a scone. A form of flat cake, baked on a griddle and popular in Scotland, and is generally made of oatmeal and takes the form of a large oatcake.

Native Americans, the Métis, and the First Nations in Canada have added bannock in their own cuisine since the 18th and 19th centuries. In western Canada, bannock is more closely associated with native culture than with its Scottish roots. This bannock consisted of white or whole wheat flour, baking powder, and water, then fried in oil (traditionally fat).

Beremeal is a whole grain flour made from bere, a variety of barley grown in northern Scotland, Orkney, and the Shetland Islands. It is commonly used in making bannocks and ale.

Oatmeal Recipes

In the old days, we all got our needed amounts of fibre, mainly because grinding and sifting flour to a fine powder would have been a lot of effort for the already over worked Celts. There is nothing wrong with whole grains in any recipe and you are going to see a lot of recipes below that are going to make it easy for you to incorporate the benefits of oats, including weight loss.

Tips for Cooking Oats:

Different types of oats require slightly different cooking methods for making hot cereal or porridge. For all types, it is best to add the oats to cold water and then cook at a simmer. The preparation of rolled oats and steel-cut oats require similar proportions using two parts water to one part oats. Rolled oats take approximately 15 minutes to cook while the steel-cut variety takes about 30 minutes. Due to their consistency, oat groats require more time and more water. Use three parts water to one part oat groats and simmer for approximately 50 minutes.

Chai Oatmeal Recipe

1 1/2 cup skim milk

1/4 tsp salt

1/4 tsp cinnamon

1/4 tsp ground coriander

1/4 tsp ground cardamom

1/4 tsp ground turmeric

drop of vanilla

2 tsp honey

3/4 cup rolled oats

2 T plain yogurt or buttermilk (optional)

Pour milk into saucepan. Add salt, cinnamon, coriander, cardamom, and turmeric. Whisk to blend. Place pan over medium heat. Just before milk comes to a boil, lower heat and let mixture simmer for about 5 minutes.

Stir in vanilla and honey and whisk until honey dissolves. Sprinkle in oats and stir once or twice. Cover pan and leave over low heat for about 8 minutes, stirring occasionally. When oatmeal has thickened to your liking, serve hot with yogurt or buttermilk.

Baked Oatmeal Recipe

2 cups oatmeal

1-1/2 teaspoon baking powder

1 cup milk

1 whole egg plus 1 egg white

1/2 cup applesauce

1/4 cup brown sugar

1/4 cup raisins

1/4 teaspoon cinnamon

1 teaspoon vanilla extract

Preheat oven to 350 degrees F, first combine the oatmeal and baking powder, then add the remaining ingredients and stir well.

Grease or spray pan and bake for 45 minutes. Stir well.

When adding oatmeal to a smoothie, you are gaining the benefits of natural raw fibre that are going to add bulk to your smoothie and help you feel full. You may taste and/or feel the soft grain of the oatmeal, but this does not deter or interfere with the deliciousness of the smoothie.

Banana Oatmeal Smoothie Recipe

1 Tbsp Instant oatmeal

1/2 cup Boiling Water

1/2 cup cold water

1 ripe Banana

1 tsp Honey

1/2 tsp Vanilla

4 Tbsp Plain yogurt

Mix boiling water and oatmeal in blender and let stand ten min, then add remaining ingredients. Blend until smooth.

Haebernes Mus, Oatmeal Mush Recipe

1 pound of Oatmeal

1 cup water

3 tablespoons Lard

1 dash Salt

In a skillet, brown the oatmeal a bit, then add water and salt. In a skillet, pan fry the resulting thick dough in the lard, where it will tear into pieces when cooking and turning.

Creamy Steel Cut Oatmeal Recipe

1 cup steel-cut oats

4 cups milk (or 2 c water, 2 c 1% milk if cutting calories)

Pinch salt

Cinnamon, to taste

1 teaspoon vanilla extract

1/3 cup dried raisins or cranberries

3 tablespoons packed brown sugar

Chopped toasted walnuts, optional

In a medium bowl, combine all ingredients. Cover and let soak in the refrigerator overnight. Transfer the oat mixture to a heavy-bottomed medium saucepan and bring to a boil over high heat. Lower the heat to maintain a gentle simmer and cook, uncovered, stirring frequently, until softened, about 10 minutes.

Serve with additional sugar and cream, if desired.

Oatmeal Almond Balls Recipe

1/3 cup of honey

2 egg whites

1/2 teaspoon ground cinnamon

1/8 teaspoon salt

1 1/2 cups uncooked quick oats

1/4 cup sliced almonds, toasted

Preheat oven to 350 degrees and combine honey, egg whites, cinnamon, and salt in large bowl; mix well. Add oats and toasted almonds; mix well. Drop by rounded teaspoonfuls onto greased or sprayed cooking sheet. Bake 12 minutes or until lightly browned and move to wire rack to cool.

Oatmeal Fruit Smoothie Recipe

1/2 cup rolled oats

2 Tbsp. wheat germ

1 cup skim milk

1 frozen banana, previously broken into chunks (before you freeze it)

8 fresh or thawed strawberries

1/2 cup fresh pineapple

1/2 teaspoon vanilla extract

Put 1st 2 ingredients in blender until oats turn to powder, then add the rest of ingredients until smooth.

Pumpkin Spiced Oatmeal Recipe

1 cup water

pinch of salt

1/3 cup quick oats

1/4 cup canned pure pumpkin

1/4 tsp cinnamon

a sprinkle of brown sugar

1 1/2 T chopped pecans or walnuts or raisins (optional)

pinch of ground nutmeg

pinch of ground cloves

Bring water to a boil and add the salt and oatmeal. Cook and stir for 90 seconds. Combine remaining ingredients in a small bowl and turn stove heat to low and stir in pumpkin mixture. Spice to taste. Serve immediately.

Homemade Instant Oatmeal Packets Recipe

3 cups oats (quick cooking works best)

pinch to 1/8 tsp of salt to taste in each bag

8 small zip-like baggies

Process ½ cup oats in a blender (or 1 cup oats in a food processor) on high until powdery. Set aside as the blender can only chop some much oatmeal at one time. Repeat with additional ½ cup oats, (or in 1 cups w/food processor).

In each baggie place 1/4 cup regular oats, 2 tablespoons powdered oats, and 1/8 teaspoon salt. Store the rest in an airtight container. To serve, empty packet into a bowl. Add 3/4 cup boiling water. Stir and let stand for 2 minutes. Adjust water amount for thicker or thinner oatmeal. Eat.

Try some of the following variations:

Sweetened Oatmeal: Add 1 T sugar Brown Sugar/Cinnamon

Oatmeal: Add 1 T brown sugar and 1/4 tsp cinnamon

Raisins and Brown Sugar: Add 1 T packed brown sugar and 1 T raisins

Apple-Cinnamon Oatmeal: Add 1 T sugar, 1/4 tsp cinnamon, & 2 T chopped dried apples

Fruit and Cream Oatmeal: Add 1 T cream and 2 T dried fruit

Wheat Germ Oatmeal: Add 2 T any kind of wheat germ

Fruit it up: with fresh or frozen, bananas or blueberries

Tropical: with shredded coconut and fresh grated mango

Nutty: with 2 T of assorted chopped nuts

Granola: add a little topping of crunchy toasted oatmeal

Maple it: with a 1/2 T of real maple syrup

Jam: a T of your favorite jam on top

And once you hit your weight loss goal, but still need to keep up the Celtic-ness of your health plan, and can add back a few non-Celtic toppings, consider whipped cream, chocolate chips, minimarshmellows, and butter and brown sugar.

Crunchy Museli

1-1/2 cups non-fat milk

1-1/4 cups Quaker Oats, Quick or Old Fashioned, uncooked

¼ cup raisins

¾ cup sweetened condensed milk

3 tablespoons lemon juice

1 medium Granny Smith apple, unpeeled, but into thin strips

2 tablespoons slivered almonds

1 teaspoon nuts and seeds, chopped

Mint leaves, if desired

Combine milk, oats, raisins and cranberries in medium bowl; cover and refrigerate overnight. In the morning, remove oats mixture from refrigerator; drain any excess liquid. Add condensed milk, lemon juice, apple, almonds and nut/seed mixture; mix well. If desired, garnish with a sprig of mint.

Maple Apple Oatmeal

3 cups apple juice

½ teaspoon ground cinnamon

¼ teaspoon salt (optional)

1-1/2 cups Oats (quick or old fashioned, uncooked)

½ cup chopped fresh or dried apple

¼ cup maple syrup

½ cup chopped nuts (optional)

In medium saucepan, bring juice, cinnamon, and salt to a boil, stir in oats, apple and syrup. Return to a boil and reduce heat to medium. Cook 1 minute for quick oats or 5 minutes for old fashioned oats or until most of juice is absorbed. Stirring occasionally. Add nuts, if desired and let stand for desired consistency.

Oatmeal Patties Recipe

1 3/4 cup boiling water

1/4 cup soy sauce

2 T vegetable oil

1 medium onion chopped or minced

1 clove garlic minced

2 cups rolled oats

3/4 teaspoon sage

2 T nutritional yeast (at health food stores)

1 egg

1/2 cup pecan meal

For casserole **gravy**:

1 can cream of mushroom soup

1/2 can milk

After oats have absorbed the boiling water, soy sauce, oil and onion, add the garlic, sage, nutritional yeast, well beaten egg, and pecan meal and mix well.

Form into patties and brown both sides well in hot greased skillet. Cover and cook until firm.

For the **casserole**:

In small bowl combine mushroom soup and milk and place the browned patties in baking dish. Cover with gravy and bake at 350 degrees until bubbly and starting to crust around the edges.

Crusts for these fruit and dessert dishes would not have the type of white flour crust that we are accustomed to today. White flour for white breads and baking did not really exist as grinding and sifting the grains would have been a lot of effort back then. Historically, white flour for baked items were generally created for those that had household staff to do such time consuming chores, such as royalty. One great old recipe for a tart crust is wholemeal flour with the addition of ground and chopped hazelnuts, which can hold a thick strained syrup of berries and honey.

Oatcakes

2 cup oatmeal

¾ cup hot water

salt

pinch of baking soda

Cook the oatmeal and the hot water into a thick porridge and add salt and a touch of baking soda. Drop by spoonfuls onto a medium hot griddle or skillet. Cook until brown on underside. The baking soda gives it a bit of a rise. Keep the griddle on low heat for best results.

Griddle Cakes, also known as Soda bread dates back to 1840 Ireland, when the baking soda, or bicarbonate of soda was available. This is a type of quick bread in which baking soda is used for leavening rather than the more common yeast. The ingredients of traditional soda bread are flour, bread soda, salt, and buttermilk. Special ingredients can be added such as raisins, egg or various forms of nuts.

The two major shapes are the loaf and the "griddle cake", or *farl* in Northern Ireland. The loaf form takes a more rounded shape and has a cross cut in the top to allow the bread to expand. The griddle cake is a more flattened type of bread. It is cooked on a griddle allowing it to take a more flat shape and split into four sections.

Soda bread eventually became a staple of the Irish diet and it is still used widely and baked in many homes on a daily or weekly basis. Tea and brown bread with pork sausages or brown bread and orange marmalade are commonly eaten for breakfast.

Old Time Oat Griddle Cakes

1/3 cup butter, melted

1 cup flour

2 1/2 tsp baking powder

1 tsp salt

1 1/2 cup quick oats

2 T sugar

2 eggs, slightly beaten.

2 cup milk

Pour the milk over the oats & let this stand 5 minutes. Stir the flour, baking powder, sugar & salt together. In another bowl, add the beaten eggs to the oat and milk mixture, plus the melted butter. Add the dry ingredients into the wet ingredients until moistened. (You could keep this in the refrigerator for several days or make as soon as possible.) Fry on griddle until brown, and serve warm.

These are thicker than usual and may take a little longer to cook than regular pancakes. Add a little more milk to thin if desired.

Oatcakes

1 lb. fine oatmeal

1/2 tsp. salt

4 tbsp. melted bacon fat or oil

8 oz boiling water

Mix together oats and salt and combine bacon fat (authentically) or vegetable oil (contemporarily) and water. Pour over the oats, quickly mix, and let sit a few minutes under a towel to cool. When cool enough to handle, knead quickly and turn onto an oatmeal dusted board. Roll as thin as possible and pinch any cracks together. Use an oat-dusted glass to cut into rounds, or make one large round and cut into triangle wedges (traditional).

Bake at 375 degrees on an ungreased baking sheet 20-30 minutes turning once, until they are gently toasted. It may be necessary to turn off the oven and leave them to dry in order to get the proper crisp texture color. Sprinkle with salt when finished.

Serve warm or cold with potted cheese. Store in an airtight container after cooled down.

Red and White Gingerbread, or "Gyngerbrede", a 1430 AD Scottish Recipe located at the National Trust of Scotland.

"Take a quart of hony, & sethe it, & skeme it clene; take Safroun, poudir Pepir & throw ther-on; take gratyd Brede & make it so chargeaunt (thick) that it wol be y-leched; then take pouder Canelle (cinnamon) & straw ther-on y-now; then make yt square, lyke as thou wolt leche yt; take when thou lechyst hyt, an caste Box (garden box) leves a-bouyn, y-stkyd ther-on, on clowys (cloves). And if thou wolt have it Red, coloure it with Saunderys (sandalwood) y-now."

Historically, Gingerbread, both red and white, was a favourite medieval sweetmeat. Home-made gingerbread could be prepared by mixing bread crumbs to a stiff paste with honey, pepper, saffron and cinnamon. Once made, it was shaped into a square, sliced and decorated with box leaves impaled on cloves.

Today's recipe version:

1 lb honey

pinch powdered saffron

1 tsp black pepper

2 tsp ground ginger

2 tsp ground cinnamon

1 lb white bread crumbs

Warm the honey until runny, then stir in the saffron and pepper. Then add the ginger and cinnamon, then mix in the bread crumbs. The mixture should be very stiff. If not, add a few more bread crumbs. Line or grease a shallow gingerbread tin and press the mixture into it with your fingers. Leave to firm up in the fridge for several hours, then remove and cut into small squares. Arrange the gingerbread on a large plate, then decorate each square with two box or small bay leaves and a whole clove stuck in the center. You can achieve an even prettier effect by gilding a few of the leaves or painting the ends of some of the cloves red.

Rough Puff Pastry

2 cup flour

1/4 tsp salt

1 stick sweet butter, chilled and cut into 1/4" bits

1/4 lb lard, prepared as the butter

4 to 6 T ice water

Sift together the flour and salt. Drop in the butter and lard, blending until the consistency of coarse meal. Pour 4 T of ice water in all at once, and gather into a ball. If dough crumbles, add ice water a tbsp at a time until it adheres together. Dust lightly with flour, wrap in waxed paper, and chill for 30 minutes.

Place pastry on lightly floured board, and press into a rectangle about 1" thick. Dust it with flour again, and roll it out into a strip about 21" long and 6" wide. Fold the strip into thirds, and roll out to the same dimensions again. Repeat this process three more times, ending with the pastry folded.

Wrap the pastry tightly in plastic wrap or a baggie, and refrigerate it for at least an hour. The pastry will keep for 3 or 4 days.

Biscuits

Ingredients:

3 cups wheat flour

1 cup flour

1 3/4 oz butter

2 eggs

1/2 tsp stevia concentrate powder

1 pkg yeast

1/2 c water, warmed

1/2 tsp vanilla

Dissolve yeast and stevia in warm water. Beat butter and eggs in separate bowl, then add flour, yeast mixture and vanilla. Let stand 40 minutes. Roll out and cut into small biscuits. Bake at 350 for 30 minutes.

Skirlie is a traditional Scottish side dish. It is eaten by itself or used as a mock stuffing.

3 oz oil for frying

2 onions, finely chopped

1/4 cup stock or water

1 3/4 cups medium oatmeal, but not rolled oats

salt and pepper to season

Heat the oil in a large frying pan. Add the onion and cook until soft and golden. Add the oatmeal and mix in well. Cook for about 5 minutes, stirring frequently. Add the stock and allow it to be absorbed by the oatmeal. Season well and serve.

Laver

Laver is Celtic for seaweed, yes that same stuff that is found on ocean beaches everywhere. Historically, every culture that has lived oceanside has had to access the ocean for available food sources. So besides the fish and shellfish, laver was very important to the food supply. Chances are you already eat some of it everyday, as it is often used as a thickener in processed foods. Seaweed was mentioned earlier, but this chapter will give you more important information as well as recipes.

The nutritional value of seaweed is high, containing an extraordinary wealth of mineral elements from the sea that can account for up to 36% of its volume. The mineral macronutrients include sodium, calcium, magnesium, potassium, chlorine, sulfur and phosphorus; the micronutrients include iodine, iron, zinc, copper, selenium, molybdenum, fluoride, manganese, boron, nickel and cobalt.

Seaweed has such a large proportion of iodine compared to dietary minimum requirements, that it is suggested as a source to obtain iodine from. The highest iodine content is found in brown algae ranging from 1500-8000 ppm (parts per million), dry rockweed from 500-1000 ppm, and red and green algae at about 100-300 ppm. Which are high when compared to any land plants. Adult requirement of iodine are recommended at 150 µg/day and easily absorbed from small quantities of seaweed. Just one gram of dried brown algae provides from 500-8,000 µg of iodine and the green and red algae (nori) provides 100-300 µg in a single gram.

The amounts of seaweed eaten as a food in Japan is often much more than 1 gram a day. The human body adapts readily to higher iodine intake, where the thyroid gland is involved in use of iodine, as it is a component of thyroid hormones. Large portions of the world population get insufficient iodine because the land, plants, and animals that serve as common dietary sources are very low in iodine. In most countries, iodine is added to table salt to assure adequate levels. China is has the largest population with a history of low iodine intake, followed by India.

Besides iodine, seaweed is one of the richest plant sources of calcium which is typically about 4-7% of dry matter. At 7% calcium, one gram of dried seaweed provides 70 mg of calcium, compared to a daily dietary requirement of about 1,000 mg. Yet this is higher than a serving of most non-milk based foods.

Protein content varies, brown algae is 5-11%, legumes are 30-40%, green algae, up to 20%, yet spirulina, a micro-alga, has a very high content being 70%. Fat content is 1-5%.

Seaweed also contains several vitamins: carotenes (provitamin A), vitamin C, B12 (which is not found in most land plants), enzymes, nucleic acids, amino acids, folic acid, minerals, trace elements, and D, E, and K vitamin complexes, oleic and alpha-linoleic acid, and high fiber.

Lignans and phytonutrients found in sea vegetables, have been shown to inhibit angiogenesis, or blood cell growth, which is the process through which fast-growing tumors gain the ability to establish secondary cancer sites. In addition, lignans have been credited with preventing estrogen synthesis in fat cells as effectively as some of the drugs used in cancer chemotherapy. In postmenopausal women, fat tissue is a primary site where estrogen is synthesized, and altered into a carcinogenic for both breast and colon cancers.

Folic acid is abundant in sea vegetables and plays a number of very important protective roles. Studies show that adequate levels of folic acid in the diet are needed to prevent certain birth defects, including spina bifida. Folic acid can also break down homocysteine, which is responsible for damaging blood vessel walls, increasing stroke risk, and cardiovascular disease. Flavoring soups and stews with sea vegetables or using them in salads is a smart strategy, especially for those dealing with atherosclerosis or diabetic heart disease.

Some sea vegetables have been shown to be unique sources of carbohydrate-like substances called fucans, which can reduce the body's inflammation. The magnesium mineral has shown to prevent migraine headaches and to reduce the severity of asthma symptoms. Magnesium may also help restore normal sleep patterns in women who are experiencing menopause. And the lignans in sea vegetables can act as very weak versions of estrogen, one of the hormones whose levels decrease during the menopausal period. For women suffering from symptoms such as hot flashes, sea vegetable's lignans may be just strong enough to ease their discomfort.

Laver is found everywhere, including the south and western shores of Wales and England and has a distinctive sea-salt taste. Traditionally, to prepare and cook Laver Bread (Bara Lawr) you gather and wash the seaweed well to remove all sand. Boil it for up to five hours until it forms a think gelatinous puree, mix it with fine oatmeal and form it into small cakes. These were fried, preferably in bacon fat, and considered excellent for breakfast. Laver sauce is begun similarly to laver bread, but without firming it with the oats.

Laver or purple laver, also known as sea lettuce, black butter, purple sea vegetable, or sloke, is scientifically known as *Porphyra umbilicalis,* but probably best known as nori, the dried sheets of seaweed used to wrap maki-type sushi.

Laver Recipes

The following recipes were created with Laver in mind. A lot of the recipes in this book could benefit from the addition of laver being added, like the soups, casserole and vegetable dishes.

Laver Crispbread

1 cup of dried nori seaweed

1 cup of ground flax meal

1 cup of steel cut oats

1 ripe tomato

1 small onion, quartered

1 grated carrot

1 red or green pepper

2 tsp fresh cilantro

¼ tsp of sea salt

1 T olive oil

1-3 T water

Soak the nori in water for a minimum of 1 hour and squeezing out the excess water with a cheesecloth or similar. Grind the flaxseed and oats with a hand grinder or coffee grinder and add to a food processor.

Remove and spread mixture evenly onto a baking sheet. Oven on the lowest temperature, about 120 degrees F. When crispbread is dry on top, turn it over and return to the oven for the other side to dry. After one hour, cut crispbread into 2" x 2" squares and allow it to continue drying in the oven.

Brown Laver Soda Bread

8 oz ground oat or barley flour

8 oz coarse ground whole meal flour

4 oz butter

1 heaping tsp baking soda

13 oz buttermilk

½ oz dried laver, chopped finely and soaked in water for 5 minutes.

Sieve the white flour, soda and salt into a bowl and cut in margarine. Add the whole meal flour and laver, then pour in buttermilk and mix (will be very moist). Pour into a greased 2 lb loaf pan and bake at 200ºC for 30-45 minutes. Cover if getting too brown.

Sauteed cabbage with Nori

1 cup roasted nori

1-2 T cooking oil

1 tsp sesame oil

1 medium sized cabbage

soy sauce

Roast the nori by placing it on an ungreased baking sheet, place in oven at 350 degrees for a few minutes, turning twice. Chop or slice the cabbage, and saute it with the roasted nori in oil until the cabbage is tender, about 5-10 minutes. Add soy sauce while cooking.

Baked Potato and Laver

4 large sized potatoes

1 medium sized red onion

butter (optional)

1 oz laver

¼ cup of cream cheese or cottage cheese

Bake the potatoes till done at 350 degrees F. Saute the finely chopped onion. Soak and rinse laver and cut into small fine pieces. Add laver to onion. Cut each baked potato in half, scoop out the potato from the half skins and combine with the butter, onion, laver and cheese, mashing all together. Return it to the half shell, broil for a couple of minutes to brown lightly, and serve.

Nori Broth

4 quarts, or 128 oz of water

1 oz of lentils

3 medium chopped onions

2 stalks chopped celery

3 medium sized potatoes

½ oz of shredded dried nori, approx. 1 cupful

1 tsp cayenne pepper

1 tsp mix herbs, your choice

Chop the onions, celery, nori and sauté in light oil for 4-5 minutes. Mix the sauteed vegetables with chopped potatoes, lentils, herbs and cayenne pepper in the water and cook for twenty minutes. Add sea salt and pepper to taste.

Atlantic Sea Soup

4 quarts or 128 oz water

½ oz of dried nori

2-3 T of soy sauce or miso

2-3 cloves of garlic

shredded fresh ginger

Simply add all ingredients to the pot, bring to a boil and simmer. Try with a sprinkle of grated cheddar and a teaspoon of cream or sour cream.

Laver Bread

4 cups prepared laver (soak cut pieces of Nori until damp but not soggy)

1 cup cut oats, quick cooking size

2-3 T oil for frying

1 lemon or 1/2 orange

salt and pepper to season to taste

Mix the Laver Bread (the soaked nori) with the oats. The mixture should be moist and hold together, but not runny, add more oats if necessary. Form into small patties and fry in oil, turning occasionally until golden brown and cooked through. Serve and sprinkle with the lemon or orange juice.

Dessert Recipes

These are good alternatives to the choices out there. And if we make these from scratch, we gain other benefits such as not adding any more chemicals to our food. Historically, desserts per se would have consisted of fruit and toasted grains and a little sugar. So if you absolutely must have some dessert, then give these a try, and freeze the rest.

Chocolate Sauce

2 oz unsweetened baking chocolate

1/2 tsp stevia concentrate powder

3/4 water

1 tsp vanilla

2 tsp arrowroot

1 TBS water

Dissolve stevia in water and then bring to a boil. Add chocolate and stir until melted. Remove from heat, add vanilla. In a separate bowl, combine 1 TBS water and arrowroot. Add to chocolate mixture and heat until thickened.

Chocolate Mousse

1-2 med. sweet potatoes cooked soft and peeled

3/4 cup unsweetened cocoa

1 cup heavy whipped cream

1 1/2 tsp of vanilla extract

1 tsp stevia liquid

Add all ingredients and blend until smooth. Adjust cocoa, stevia and/or vanilla to suit taste. Add walnuts, almonds or carob chips for a variation.

Lemon Ice Cream

1/2 tsp stevia concentrate powder

1 cup milk

1 cup whipped cream

1/4 cup lemon juice

1/2 tsp lemon concentrate

Mix stevia, milk and cream. Stir until mixed thoroughly and stevia is dissolved. Cover with stretch wrap and freeze for 1 1/2 hours. Add juice and extract. Beat thoroughly, cover and return to freezer. Wait 2 hours and then beat again. Remove and whip 1/2 hour before serving.

Vanilla Ice Cream

1/2 tsp stevia concentrate powder

1 cup milk

dash of salt

1 cup half and half

2 cups whipped cream

1 1/2 tsp vanilla

While stirring, scald milk. Dissolve stevia in milk, remove from heat, add remaining ingredients. Cover and place in fridge until cooled then freeze.

Must Have Fruit Popsicles

fresh or frozen fruit

water

stevia

We made these as kids. Simply put your fruit and a little real fruit juice into a blender and puree. Pour into the popsicle tray and add the little sticks. Enjoy.

Fruit Snow Cones

Not everyone has a ice shaver, but if you do, or want to get one, I think it would come in very handle for recipes just like this one.

1 cup fresh or frozen fruit

stevia to sweeten

fresh snow or shaved ice

Blend fruit in blender, add sweetener, and pour over ice.

Chocolate Fluff

1/2 cup whipping cream

1/4 teaspoon vanilla

1/4 teaspoon white stevia powder

1 teaspoon unsweetened dark cocoa powder

Whip the cream, vanilla and stevia in a bowl until stiff peaks form, then stir in the cocoa powder and enjoy.

Carob Chocolate Pudding

1/3 cup flour

1/2 cup cocoa

1/2 cup carob

1/2 tsp stevia concentrate powder

1/4 tsp salt

1 3/4 cups skim milk

1 oz unsweetened chocolate

1 T butter

In a saucepan, combine flour, cocoa, carob, stevia and salt. Gradually add milk and whisk until smooth. Place over medium heat and stir constantly. Once hot, add chocolate and butter, stir until well blended and thick. Pour into container(s) and chill.

Chocolate chip cookies

1/2 cup cashew or nut butter

1/4 cup oil

1/2 cup apple butter

1/3 tsp powdered Stevia extract

1/2 tsp Stevia concentrate

1 tsp vanilla extract

1 cup oatmeal flour

1/4 tsp baking soda

1/4 tsp salt

1/2 cup chocolate chips OR carob ships

Preheat oven to 375 degrees, grease a cookie sheet. Cream the cashew butter and oil together in a mixing bowl. Add the apple butter, Stevia extract, Stevia concentrate, and vanilla extract. Combine flour, baking soda, and salt together, add to wet ingredients. Stir in chocolate or carob chips.

Spoon onto cookie sheet and flatten with palm of hand. Bake 12 - 15 minutes, makes 16. Eat a couple and freeze the rest.

Raspberry Sherbet

2 cups plain yogurt

1/4 cup milk

1/2 cup unsweetened raspberry juice blend concentrate (thawed)

1 T orange juice concentrate or blend (thawed)

1 tsp vanilla extract

3/4 tsp. powdered Stevia extract

1 banana (optional)

Blend all ingredients together in a blender until smooth. Pour into the container of the ice cream machine and process according to directions. You can also substitute the yogurt for 12 oz of silken tofu, and up the milk portion to 1 cup. You can vary this recipe by using other types of fruit concentrates.

Stevia Equivalency Chart

Sugar	Green Stevia Powder	Stevia Liquid
1 cup	1.5 T	1 tsp
1 T	1/8-¼ tsp	6-9 drops
1 tsp	1 tsp pinch	2-4 drops

Apple-Oat Bread Pudding

4 large dessert apples

3 oz fresh brown bread crumbs

1 oz oatmeal

2.5 oz melted butter

6 oz natural sugar OR 2 oz sugar and 1/2 tsp liquid stevia

1 tsp ground cinnamon

1/4 tsp ground cloves

juice of 1 lemon

Peel, core and slice the apples. Mix the breadcrumbs and butter. Combine the sugar and spices. To assemble, place a third of the crumbs in a round ovenproof dish, top with half of the apples then half of sugar. Squeeze over half of the lemon juice then continue layering: a third crumbs, half apples, half sugar, remaining lemon juice then final third crumbs.

Cover with foil and bake at 180C/350F for about 45 minutes or until apples are just tender, then remove foil, increase heat to 200C/400F for a further 15 minutes or so, until browned. Eat warm with thick cream.

Rough Puff Pastry

8 oz flour

4 oz butter

1/2 tsp salt

few drops of lemon juice

cold water

Sieve the flour and salt into a bowl; add the lemon juice and the butter broken into pieces the size of a walnut; add sufficient cold water to bind the ingredients together.

Turn on to a floured board, and roll the pastry into a long strip. Fold it in three, and press the edges together. Half turn the pastry, rib it with the rolling pin to equalize the air in it, and again roll it into a strip. Fold in three and repeat this until the pastry has had four rolls, folds and half-turns. It is then ready for use.

Drink Recipes

First and foremost, water must be at the top of our list when it comes to the liquids that we drink. There were no slurpees and ice cappuccinos back in the historical days. It would have been water, and more water, then perhaps teas made with herbs. Granted there may have been more Scotch Whisky some days, but for the most part, it was water.

But we are not used to good plain water these days. So the next best thing here is to turn to water up a notch and thus guarantee that we will be more likely to drink it. Remember in the Contemporary Additions Chapter we covered the plant Stevia. This sweet leaf plant is going to save any dieter from cheating. We can now have all the sweet drinks we want and be happy knowing that we aren't adding any sugar or chemicals to our bodies.

Considering watering down any fruit juices. Often citric acid is added making them a little too tart, and these juices are just as good watered down. And learn to carry a water bottle with you everywhere.

Fennel Tea can be made with one-half teaspoon of crushed seeds per one cup of boiling water.

Consider chewing on a few fennel seeds when the need to overeat is calling.

Warm Oatmeal Protein Drink Recipe

1 cup filtered water

1/3 cup quick oats

1 T maple syrup

1 scoop vanilla protein powder

1 shake of ground cinnamon

Heat the water to a near boil, add oats and let stand for 5 minutes.

Place in a blender, and add maple syrup and protein powder. Blend until smooth. Pour into a mug and shake cinnamon on top.

Kale Juice Recipes

Enjoy the many health benefits of kale with the following juice recipes:

-5 kale leaves, 3 carrots, 1 orange

-6 kale leaves, 1 celery stalk, 1/2 pineapple, 1" ginger root

-2 cups kale, 1 cup spinach, 2 cups parsley, 3 celery stalks, 1 cucumber, small amount of garlic and/or ginger (optional)

Ginger ale

3 1/2 cup water

3/4 cup peeled and chopped ginger root

2 T vanilla

1 T lemon extract

1/4 tsp stevia powder

carbonated or sparkling water

Rapidly boil ginger root in water for 10 minutes. Strain and place liquid in a jar. Stir in vanilla, lemon and stevia. Cool and store in the refrigerator.

Lemon-Lime-Ade

This is a great combination of lemons and limes, but you could also make this with all lemon juice, all lime juice, or orange or grapefruit juice. Makes about 3 cups concentrate.

1 lemon

1 lime

1 teaspoon white powdered stevia

3 cups water

Squeeze the juice from the lemon and the lime into a measuring cup. Add the stevia and stir to dissolve. Pour into a storage bottle, add the water, and stir or shake to blend and store in fridge.

When preparing your drink, mix it 50/50 with water or sparkling water and ice.

Iced Coffee

4 teaspoons instant coffee (I use organic decaf)

3/4 teaspoon white powdered stevia

2 cups water

cream to taste (optional)

Dissolve the instant coffee in 1/2 cup of hot water and add the the 1 1/2 cups of cold water. Add the stevia and chill. Pour over crushed ice and enjoy.

Lemonade

1 pint or 32 oz bottle or container of water, add

¼ cup of lemon juice, natural bottled variety or from fresh lemons

1 dropper full of liquid stevia.

Pour over ice, or drink as is. Check the equivalency chart for Stevia measurements.

Iced Tea

Basically, you will start with the Lemonade recipe above. Make tea with one or two teabags in one cup of water and add this to your Lemonade recipe.

Coffees

There are so many specialty coffees out there, making coffee even nicer to drink these days. Check the coffee aisle for the assorted flavors and caffeine contents. Make some hot coffee in the morning, turn it off, and drink it with ice and vanilla and stevia in the afternoon.

Root Beer

3 T sarsaparilla root (about 1/2 ounce)

1 T licorice root

1 qt purified water

2-3 tsp dried Stevia leaf

2 qt carbonated water

Simmer the sarsaparilla and licorice root in the quart of water for about 45 minutes. Do not boil as this may cause it to turn bitter. Add the Stevia leaf or teabags and simmer for 15 minutes longer.

Strain the plant material out and return the pan to the burner. Simmer on very low until liquid is reduced to half. Remove from heat and strain through a cheesecloth. You will be left with about 12 ounces of concentrate. Chill in refrigerator.

For a glass of fresh naturally made root beer, add two ounces of concentrate to 10-12 ounces carbonated water. Add Stevia extract to taste, if more sweetener is desired.

Nettle tea

Nettle, also known as Stinging Nettle, and a wild growing plant with health benefits. It does make a bitter tea if used alone, so add it to other teas.

Folklore

Interesting facts about things Celtic

In Derbyshire, the juice of the Dandelion stalk is applied to remove warts. The milky latex has been used as a mosquito repellent and the roots can be used as a dye.

Externally, onions have been used to heal blisters and boils and is a component in the medicinal cream Mederma.

In India, fennel seeds are used as an after-dinner breath freshener and digestive.

Dandelion Barometers (it's true!):

"The dandelion is an excellent barometer, one of the commonest and most reliable. It is when the blooms have seeded and are in the fluffy, feathery condition that its weather prophet facilities come to the fore. In fine weather the ball extends to the full, but when rain approaches, it shuts like an umbrella. If the weather is inclined to be showery it keeps shut all the time, only opening when the danger from the wet is past." Source: "Camping For Boys," by H.W. Gibson

Rosemary, For a tonic against headaches put some sprigs into a teapot add hot water strain and serve.

Daily Menu Examples

In the course of planning your week of meals, make larger batches, as they will last for days in the fridge, or you can freeze them and take out as needed. Make a plan, because unless you like spending time in the kitchen, all that cooking, cleaning and creating meals is one of the reasons we don't eat properly. Being creative meal-wise at the end of the day is frustrating if you are tired or hungry or family is wanting to eat NOW. Make a plan and add just enough organization to be prepared for those busy or tired meal times.

Day 1

In the morning, make 1 cup of oatmeal (1/3 cup oats, 2/3 cup water).

Make a batch of Vegetarian Cock-a-leekie Soup.

Make a liter or quart of Lemonade with Stevia and drink throughout the day. Make another quart if desired.

Breakfast

1/4 cup of oatmeal, warm or hot, with healthy toppings or plain,

1 egg, cooked any way, keep the oil amount low or fry in water,

1/2 sliced tomato,

1/2 sliced apple, plain or with dash of cinnamon.

tea or coffee

Lunch

1/4 cup of oatmeal, plain or a little bit of toppings,

1/2 cup of yogurt, all natural with probiotics,

1/2 cup of fruit, any kind,

1 bowl full of your Cock-a-Leekie Soup,

carrot sticks, one carrots worth, could use yogurt for dip.

Try a little of yogurt and oatmeal on each spoonful.

Mid afternoon snack

Choices: 1/4 cup of oatmeal, bowl of soup, 1/4 cup of fruit, a boiled egg.

Dinner

1 bowl full of soup,

cabbage stir fry, as much as you want,

protein source such as 4 oz of seasoned and baked chicken, fish, or meat

for dessert, berries/fruit with a little cream or yogurt

still hungry? you still have 1/4 cup of oatmeal. Try it cold with a little honey drizzled on top.

Day 2

oven toast 1/2 cup of uncooked rolled oats

make a batch of cream of celery soup

Breakfast

1/4 cup of cottage cheese,

sprinkled with 1/8 cup of toasted oats,

sprinkled with honey,

1/4 cup of fruit,

Mix fruit, cottage cheese together, then add oats and honey.

tea or coffee

lunch

bowl full of cream of celery soup

cheese stuffed figs

veggies sticks with walnut dressing

snack

choices: 1/4 cup of yogurt with 1/8 cup of toasted oats, 1/4 cup fruit with 1/8 cup of toasted oats.

Dinner

bowl full of cream of celery soup

Potch Erfyn, cooked turnips and potatoes mashed together

4 oz of baked and seasoned salmon

Dessert

1/4 cup of the toasted oats with 1/4 cup of blueberry sauce.

Now it is time to take the great information contained in this book and let it lead you to a healthier place. Those pounds will fall off, your health will improve, and in a few short weeks, you will be seeing a new person in the mirror. A happier and thinner person. The person that you naturally are meant to be.

About the Author

Meet Breanne Findlay, an herbalist, aromatherapist, author, writer, and natural-products expert who has spent years bringing natural living to others through websites, authoring three health books and how-to videos, and teaching classes. Breanne brings her nutritional expertise, along with her Celtic roots, to create a health-restoring book that incorporates the culture and tradition of Celtic foods.